MW00436075

The Little Book
for Alzheimer's Caregivers

Celia Koudele

© 2014 Celia Koudele
All Rights Reserved.

No part of this publication may be reproduced, stored in a retrieval system, or transmitted, in any form or by any means, electronic, mechanical, photocopying, recording, or otherwise, without the written permission of the author.

First published by Dog Ear Publishing
4010 W. 86th Street, Ste H
Indianapolis, IN 46268
www.dogearpublishing.net

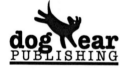

ISBN: 978-1-4575-2912-2

This book is printed on acid-free paper.

Printed in the United States of America

Dedication

I would like to dedicate this book to
My Mom, My Aunt and My Nana,
who suffered from Alzheimer's disease.

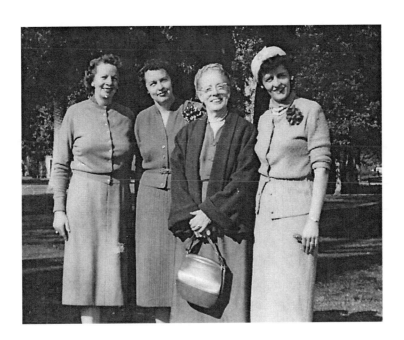

"It is only Memory Loss"

So I asked my grandchildren "What is a Memory?"

"A thing a long, long time ago that you remember, like if you went to the park yesterday you would still remember it today.

(From 8 year old grandson Aiden)

"When you remember something good for a really long time."

(From 7 year old granddaughter Wren)

"Memory is keeping something in your mind, for a long time."

(From 7 year granddaughter Carson)

We have good, bad, and idle memories. Hopefully we all make good memories we can store and then retrieve when we need them. Maybe daily memory loss is only a symptom of the too many things in our life to remember! It doesn't always mean you have dementia.

Acknowledgements

I felt compelled to write this book, hoping someone out there could benefit from the knowledge and experience I gained from caring for my family and working with the Alzheimer's Association. There is so much to know!

But without the support of my spouse and the wonderful editing of my daughter-in-law Desiree, I would never have the courage to write a book. Thanks to them and my friends who also read my book, encouraged me, and made valuable suggestions; Diane, Ginger, Bob, Ginny, Evelyn, Candi, and Marsha

People ask me when I tell them about my mom, grandmother and aunt having this disease if I'm afraid I will get it also. (I have some of the other risk factors too)

The answer is <u>Yes</u>.

Table of Contents

INTRODUCTION

My story

I'm passionate about Alzheimer's disease. I want to help others learn about it, to recognize it, and deal with it. It is my past, present and probably my future. I share your journey in many ways. My mother, grandmother and an aunt all died from this disease. My mother died at 85 years, my aunt at 79 years and my grandmother at 77 years. They all share genetic traits but the course of the disease and type of Dementia were different, for all of them. I worked at the Alzheimer's Association of Central and Western Kansas, Wichita, Ks for 9 years and have continued to volunteer there. My job was to talk with over 60 families a month with questions, problems, tears, and their exhaustion dealing with Dementia. I have heard stories about the horror of the disease, the fear, frustration, pain, denial and hopelessness. I think I can help, because I experienced many of those feelings caring for my Mom and seeing my grandmother decline.

My mother was well educated, (she had two college degrees) she traveled the world, lived on a farm, was very conscious of eating healthy because her mom was a nurse and she reached out to help everyone. She wrote two books and could converse on anything. Mom was my best friend!

There are no easy answers, and many of you just want someone to listen who understands. I have no fancy titles, but I've shared a similar journey. Before my time has come, and I don't remember the things I learned from others and on my own, I would hope these words could help someone!

This book is solely for the purpose of helping families with Alzheimer's. You as caregivers don't have time for lots of reading. You need ideas to try today. It helps to have an understanding of why normal interactions don't work with an Alzheimer's person. When families are in the middle of Alzheimer's disease, they are so busy dealing with the everyday problems, they lose sight of the big picture.

Let's go down this journey together. In the following pages I will share my ideas for problems you may have every day and how to keep your perspective through the disease.

Celia Koudele, BA, MA

CHAPTER 1

The basics of Alzheimer's disease

"It is only memory loss?"

"Don't you worry you will get Alzheimer's?"

"Did I do the right thing by placing my mom in a nursing home, I feel so guilty?"

"I am afraid he might hurt me."

"My wife is talking to ghosts in the basement".

"I just can't take it anymore, my wife is crazy and now she is speaking another language!"

"The medicine isn't helping, now what?"

"Who are you and what am I doing here?"

These are the cries from families with Alzheimer's. Some are sure there must be a "cure" somewhere, some caregivers become exhausted and then become ill, few understand the disease and many just want courage and ideas to face another day with this deadly disease.

This book is for all of those families, drowning with the symptoms and the realities of Alzheimer's or another type of Dementia.

Alzheimer's is a progressive, degenerative, neurological disease. It gradually destroys brain cells and

affects a person's memory, ability to make judgments, communicate and carry out basic daily activities.

It is the ultimate thief. It steals memories, independence, control and eventually life! Yes, you can die from Alzheimer's.

Someone is diagnosed with Alzheimer's every 69 seconds; there are over 5.4 million people with this disease. It is the only one of the top 10 causes of death in the U.S. without an identified means to prevent it, cure it or even slow its progression. There is lots of research to prove that effective care and support for the caregiver and person with Alzheimer's improves the "quality of life" for them both. This book is for you! There are many books about Alzheimer's some with a clinical view, others focus solely on the caregiving for their family member and some have a specific approach to dealing with people who have dementia.

Most everyone knows someone with Alzheimer's or is related to someone with Alzheimer's disease. But families rarely tell the public or discuss with others about the true devastation of this disease. Sometimes "memory loss" is the easiest symptom. Every family and person is different.

There are over 50 types of dementia, Alzheimer's accounts for about 70 per cent. For the purpose of this book we will use "dementia" & Alzheimer's" interchangeably. Some other types include Picks, Parkinson's, Multi-infarct, Huntington's, Cruetzfeldt-Jakob (mad cow) and Lewy body

Most dementias are very similar. However, the parts of the brain that are affected differ. They can lose the ability to speak; they can have hallucinations; and can talk, but do not have the ability to comprehend the conversation. Other people with different types won't lose their memory until later in the disease. People have told me their loved one suddenly became extroverts and made friends with everyone in the grocery store. Some seemed to pick a family member to be angry with all the time but become too mellow to want to do anything.

This book is to give an "overall" guide to the symptoms and problems dealing with dementias. It is meant as a quick handy guide with ideas to use right now.

We all may forget part of our day, but a person with dementia forgets the whole day; we forget our keys, but a person with dementia forgets what the keys are used for; we can usually decipher things with directions; but this disease makes it gradually impossible to do that.

The individual who is sick often doesn't remember they have a disease. Families say "they don't think anything is wrong with them." Who wants to remember they have a fatal disease that will take their dignity, change their behavior, let them forget the people they love and may turn them into an angry person no one wants to be near?

Unfortunately, spouses and family members try to reason with the confused person about driving, living alone and going to the doctor. All of this doesn't work because the affected person often can't make logical thought. (One of the warning signs)

There is lots of research on dementia. But currently there are only a few drugs that help some people with the symptoms. People say "Isn't there some drugs for that?" Yes, but currently none can even offer hope for a cure. Most drugs deal with the depression, psychotic behavior, anxiety and try to help with activities of living.

Yes, Alzheimer's can be genetic. If a person is diagnosed with Alzheimer's before 65 years, one out of two children will likely also develop the disease.

It used to be, the only way to know if someone had Alzheimer's was with an autopsy. New methods of diagnosing (brain scan, mini mental test, blood work and family history) can be 90 - 92 percent accurate. Many families don't go to the doctor soon enough. Some of the current medications work best in the early part of the disease. That being said, if they don't have long-term care insurance or health insurance, a company may not cover them once they have a diagnosis. Durable Power of Attorney for Health Care and Financial are very important also.

Many people think this is "an old person's disease". But tell that to the 44 year-old who died from a type of dementia, leaving a 10year-old at home. What about nursing homes that are not prepared or trained to care for 50 year old dementia patient? How does the spouse of a 50 year old hold a job and take care of her sick husband who needs more and more care?

Denial

Families become frustrated, angry and often just give up trying to help if they suspect there is a problem. The loved one or spouse may become very defensive if any symptoms are mentioned. Then there are the members of the family who see "nothing wrong" with Mom or Dad. Denial is comforting. If they don't admit anything is wrong, they don't have to physically do anything to help, financially offer to pay for help or emotionally deal with the fact that a parent may have a disease that makes them "crazy!"

Denial is a loss for everyone, the person who is sick loses a chance to interact and make memories with friends and family while they still know them and are able to enjoy their company. It is a loss for others because this is a progressive, degenerative disease, and often by the time family and friends accept it, the person they know and love is gone. Life has no guarantees; each day is different and just because life is busy with jobs and kids, it doesn't mean life stands still for others we love.

We can all pretend, "They don't have Alzheimer's," "It is not that bad, she sounds normal on the phone" or "I am too busy or too far away to help." **Everyone loses when we deny there is a problem!** It could be something simple like dehydration, because older people often don't drink enough water, but by denying there are any symptoms your loved one suffers confusion and other symptoms when there might be an easy fix.

My mom was deathly sick twice in her life. As we began to notice her searching for words, forgetfulness, and unsteady gait it was easy to blame the earlier sicknesses. We knew her mother had died from this disease, but mom was so vibrant and dynamic, how could she have Alzheimer's?

Families often say that Alzheimer's is such an "awful" disease. So are there some GOOD diseases? Ask that of a child with leukemia, or someone with breast cancer. The difference is usually that with most diseases there is some medicine or treatment that might be a cure. There is none for Alzheimer's or dementia and some researchers aren't even sure what causes it. In the beginning of the disease, people suffering look normal, and on a "good" day can act normal. But day by day the brain robs them of a personality and memories that make them unique. The deterioration of the brain causes memory loss and can cause disorientation, angry agitated behavior, inappropriate behavior, paranoia, hallucinations, fear of bathing and sexual problems; just to name a few. Eventually it robs their bodies also, and they begin to have problems with depth perception, walking, finding words, weight loss or weight gain and swallowing. **Unlike other diseases, it first takes their mind and personality, then their body.**

The "blessings" of Alzheimer's are that it is a slowly progressing disease. This usually allows families and friends to adjust to the fact that this is a disease, not just a group of symptoms, learn about it and enjoy the person that is still there. Each day and sometimes hour is different for people with Alzheimer's. That is why it is hard for a family to all be on the same page as they each see a different person.

The media is only beginning to talk about Alzheimer's disease. We have no survivors to champion our cause, President Reagan with Alzheimer's has long been mostly forgotten and no details are given about how hard it is for the famous basketball coach Pat Summit to live every day with this disease.

Many people are ashamed if their family member suffers from this disease. Their loved one might say inappropriate things like cuss words, or dress with several layers of clothes. It is a secret. Money can buy the best care in the world, but it doesn't stop the symptoms of the disease. It doesn't stop the pain of watching someone you love become helpless like a child. This disease happens; regardless of rich, poor, young, old, Caucasian, African-American, President or dock worker. Nothing can stop it.

My thoughts:

From my experience with my mom and others, I think this message reflects how they may feel.

Speak a little slower*. We all don't process information as fast as we used to. Maybe their hearing aid isn't working or there is a lot of background noise.*

Accept your loved one's answers*. They may be protecting the feelings of someone else or their own memory. Never argue with your loved one. They may still know how to "push your buttons" but back away.*

Help your loved one retain their dignity*. Others don't need to know their capabilities or shortcomings*

We all need to be our brother's keeper*. Your loved one may just be having a bad day or is exhausted.*

Be patient*. Can you imagine the turmoil in your loved one's mind? They may be angry because forgetfulness can make us appear stupid.*

Give them a choice*. They may have forgotten the options or are too tired to make a decision. We all need the question patiently repeated some days.*

CHAPTER 2

How can this book help?

The goal is to help families make sense of Alzheimer's disease. There are reasons for diagnosis, for communicating differently, for making the home safe, for keeping a journal, for awareness about medications and mostly to help you be the best CAREGIVER and helper you can be.

If some ideas help you cope one more day with the frustrating symptoms of this disease, it is worth it. Often I was in tears and desperate, as I had no ideas how to deal with each new symptom or behavior of this disease. Who could I ask, who could really understand the emotional journey of it?

The Alzheimer's Association has a 24/7, 1-800-272-3900 helpline and there are many blogs and support groups online to help families. Support groups are not just places to complain, but to gain ideas about what worked for others!

Sometimes as families are so busy just putting out the day to day "fires" of this disease; they lose sight of the bigger picture. We can't change the behavior of a person with Alzheimer's disease, but we can change their medication and the way we approach and talk with them.

It is important to help the person with Alzheimer's retain who they are! They are probably someone's spouse, father, mother, grandfather, grandmother, uncle or aunt, and had a great job. They made a difference in the world, and we all like to be reminded we are important to someone and we did a good job.

Fear can be a big part of the disease.

For the person with Alzheimer's disease they worry about such things as: Will I forget who you are? When will I no longer be me, but an old confused person in a wheelchair? I don't want my family to remember me confused. Don't tell anyone I have this disease. It is rarely the fear of dying or being ill, it is the fear of not remembering who loves us.

Spouses, of those who have Alzheimer's suffer in a different way. They lose a companion, often a sexual partner, someone to help with life decisions like buying a car. They lose dreams of traveling together as they age and they accept a job of caregiving that neither may be prepared for. Each day the person with dementia may be right in front of them, and yet a little more of their loved one is gone.

Watching a parent become ill is scary in a different way. Parents always told us what to do, how do we prepare for role reversal? There is no EASY way to watch parents become ill. Sometimes they don't want to share what you need to know to help them on this journey. Often there is a real struggle for control. Children want to let them be independent and make their own decisions. Remember because of the disease, they can become a danger to themselves or others.

My thoughts:

- *Choose your battles. You can't be everything to everyone. Set priorities, seek help and choose what you can do today.*

- *Accept the change.*

- *Decide to do what you can, when you can, with smiles and laughter. Attitude can affect everyone.*

- *Some days it is OK to cry. There are so many aspects of this disease that are overwhelming. There are days the "dragon" wins! Tomorrow is another day and it will be different.*

- *Celebrate each smile, memory or laugh. We all want to leave this world recalling the "happy" times of our life. Children, vacations, silly mistakes, weddings, reunions or parties. Recall them today.*

CHAPTER 3

Warning signs

"The doctor just changed her medicine".

"She is just getting over a cold".

"He seems really tired lately".

We all have excuses for not noticing or accepting the warning signs of dementia! The days that are good make us forget about the suspicions we had before.

Rarely is it a big thing that sends families for a diagnosis. Sometimes being in the hospital, the staff picks up on it. Surgery for older people (the stress and drugs) can cause a type of dementia that in time disappears with recovery. Patients in a hospital can also have delirium which is more related to drugs and pain, but is not dementia or Alzheimer's.

It is usually the little things that get families to the Doctor. It can be simple things like searching for words or not being able to make decisions at a restaurant or at home. Maybe it is unusual things in places in her cupboards, spending money on the same thing like four bottles of olive oil, or he seems restless and not able to finish tasks. Their sense of "time" can become noticeable. Maybe you called and told them you would be there in an hour, but you arrive to discover they have been sitting on the porch waiting in the heat since you talked on the phone because they no longer can judge ten minutes or one hour.

Start by keeping a journal. Write down the little things you see. Little things don't count, but frequent and many little things helps you see the bigger picture.

Develop an awareness of their surrounding:

Do pots and pans have several burn spots?

Does it look like the bills are being paid (subtle discussions can help)?

Does there seem to be more clutter everywhere?

Are their medicine boxes orderly and it looks like they are taking them?

Look at the car, are there new dents?

Physical and Behavioral Signs

Weight Loss- Alzheimer's people will cover all these problems as long as possible, sometimes for years! They can blame any of these issues on something. My mom used to say "I've just not been hungry." When the truth is they have forgotten to eat, they don't remember where the food is or can't remember how to run the microwave.

Agitation or anger- Maybe your loved one has always had an "unpleasant" personality. You blame it on old age, or the pain of arthritis. But maybe the disease has added to the problem?

Speech problems-How often do we forget a name or face and we need help remembering? We use the wrong word for something, but continue talking so no one notices.

<u>Word Finding</u>-Doesn't everyone say," You know, that thing we use to make cake with?" But frequent looking for words is not normal.

<u>Paranoia</u>- People who live alone often thinks someone is in their house stealing from them, as they misplace things. But sometimes they think someone has stolen valuables and begins blaming all family members. Unless there is a reason to believe there is a theft, it can be a symptom of the disease.

<u>Hallucinations</u>-A mirror can be scary for someone suffering from hallucinations. They may not recognize themselves in a mirror, and so are afraid of every mirror.

<u>Inappropriate Sexual Behavior</u>- Alzheimer's disease can make people lose their inhibitions. They lose the ability to remember what is socially acceptable. So this may mean they wear inappropriate clothes, take off their clothes and use profane language. This can be symptom of the disease.

<u>Incontinence</u>- Incontinence can become more of an issue the older we get. But people with Alzheimer's have difficulty with thought processes. They can't figure out how to get help or deal with the problem.

All these symptoms don't happen to all Alzheimer's people. They definitely don't all happen in the early stages.

Compare notes with other family members. Families who are involved subconsciously see things. Maybe a sister has a "strange" conversation with Mom but doesn't share with the sister who also had a "strange" visit with Mom.

Early diagnosis

It is important to get a diagnosis as soon as possible.

Current medications are most effective in the early stages of the disease. An early diagnosis will also help you determine if there is another cause for the behavior you are seeing, such as a brain tumor.

There could be an easy solution like not enough potassium, sodium, diabetes, thyroid imbalance, low levels of Vitamin B or D. Blood tests will determine most of these, but sometimes you have to ask about Vitamin D and B levels. (It is common for Alzheimer's people to lack vitamin B because their body has lost the ability to absorb it naturally.) Lots of new research suggests how important Vitamin D is for our system to work. In climates where winter prevents much exposure to natural sunlight it is really important.

People wonder WHY we need a diagnosis. They are just old and senile. Because maybe they are NOT! Don't consider an online test, drugstore smell test or clinic that offers a "quick" memory test. People sometimes take these and then become convinced they are fine. When it could be they have something else physically wrong that is just beginning.

All old people don't get Alzheimer's disease! Just ask some of those who are over 100.

Most tests are simple, and what a relief for the person and family if it is an "easy" fix. Sometimes people with dementia are relieved to finally know what is wrong. Each day is precious and ignorance is rarely bliss.

Things to consider in the early stages

Living alone can be dangerous with memory loss.

People with memory problems can be vulnerable. Telemarketers can call and they send money, but forget because of short term memory loss, so they send money again. They forget to pay bills, but families don't know because they "seemed" fine, so no one tactfully asked. (In my experiences in working with families, one family's mom was going to be evicted for not making house payments. Luckily someone called her daughter to make sure she knew.) Another lady had a $10,000 bill to the Home Shopping Network, because as soon as she hung up, she forgot she ordered and ordered again!

Medication can pose another danger to those alone. Taking the right medication at the right time can be confusing for all of us. But just a little confusion can make filling those pill boxes, overwhelming. Worse yet, they may forget all together. Sometimes if it has been a long day, they think it is the next day, and take that medication too.

There is a fine line between allowing people the dignity to live their life as they choose, being independent, and turning a blind eye to potential problems.

Rarely does anyone want to admit or tell someone they think there is a problem.

There are over 100 ways to compensate for symptoms of Alzheimer's. The unknown is usually scarier than what we know. Sometimes people go to the doctor for other symptoms like heart disease, cancer, or joint problems and the doctor notices other problems.

Would you make them go to the doctor for high blood pressure, a lump, or trouble breathing? Alzheimer's is a DISEASE. It has different symptoms, it creeps up like a silent killer, but life isn't over because of a diagnosis. Maybe a good friend or family member needs to encourage them to go to doctor for symptoms. But even the person with memory loss or other issues needs to write them down; if they are able and admit they don't feel well. Doctors don't know how to help if they just tell them they are more forgetful. (See alz.org for a checklist to take to doctor.)

It is exhausting to compensate for the symptoms that gradually begin to appear.

Usually the person with the disease is aware something is wrong. But they don't want to have their independence threatened by sharing what they are feeling. It takes a lot of energy to cover all the symptoms. Paying attention to others when they don't remember what the conversation is about is exhausting! Often the person with symptoms begins to withdraw, so they don't have to deal with the confusion of the world.

Forgetting doctor appointments, can be explained when they say they forgot to write it down, or they heard the receptionist wrong. Not being ready when the daughter came to pick them up can be excused by "I thought it was another day."

Every day that a person with Alzheimer's and their family ignores that there is a problem, is a day out of their life!

Know the 10 Warning signs of Dementia:
(from Alzheimer's Association)

1. Memory loss that disrupts daily life.

2. Challenges in planning or solving problems.

3. Difficulty completing familiar tasks at home, work or leisure.

4. Confusing time and place.

5. Trouble understanding visual images and spatial relationship.

6. New problems with words in speaking or writing.

7. Misplacing things and losing ability to retrace steps.

8. Decreased or poor judgment.

9. Withdrawal from work or social activities.

10. Changes in mood and personality.

My thoughts:

- *Start with a journal. No one can remember all the little things that can be symptoms. Be aware of physical signs, even dress and appearance. A person who was a classy dresser can begin wearing soiled clothes. Be aware if they have been falling.*

- *Early diagnosis is the key! But be sure accurate tests are performed before accepting diagnosis.*

- *Living alone can be dangerous-be aware of dangers.*

- *Rarely does a person admit they could have symptoms of Alzheimer's.*

- *It is exhausting! No wonder they seem so tired.*

CHAPTER 4

Understanding behaviors associated with Alzheimer's

Sometimes it helps us if we can understand why people with Alzheimer's behave the way they do.

People who have Alzheimer's usually have good long-term memory, because the events of their past are now vividly and emotionally stored in their brains. However, they often can't learn new things. They can't store, recall or reflect on what you just said, or what they said, so they **repeat it over and over**. Their brains begin to short circuit. Often people with Alzheimer's can give you details of their first car, but rarely tell you where you all went to dinner last night! Accept whatever answer they give, and if you really need something more specific, ask later.

Unmet Physical Needs.

For example, we all need to feel safe in our own home, but if the disease has affected our ability to determine if we are safe, we may become paranoid. Be aware of physical needs that they express with difficult behavior like yelling, agitation or displays of rejection. They may only need to find the bathroom or are frustrated because they are hungry and can't find food. People with this disease can become obsessive compulsive, hoarders, dress in dirty clothes or become an extrovert in the grocery store. Remember that one of the warning signs is: CHANGES IN PERSONALITY.

It is tempting to respond abruptly or reach for pills when you can't reason with someone. During times like this it is important to be patient and try to find another way to achieve the behavior you are seeking. Practice thinking outside the box is good for all of us! Consider if they are in pain, or haven't been sleeping well, or maybe even have a sinus infection. The disease often makes them unable to process solutions to simple problems! Sometimes people with Alzheimer's can "cuss" or strike out at family or friends. They don't know how else to tell you something is WRONG.

TIP: Can you imagine being so confused you don't know where the refrigerator is or remember to drink water? If any of us get dehydrated it can cause confusion. Subtly remind them how important it is to drink water and even leave some bottles of water around. As we age, we have a diminished thirst response and coupled with side effects of medication that we take (diuretics), it can cause further dehydration.

Unmet Emotional Needs

Emotional needs can be seen if they are sitting in their chair all day, they don't do, see, or remember things to do that made their life complete. Many people suffer from depression and that explains the behavior. Sometimes they are just "bored" and can't think of anything else to do, so they become restless and pace. Being with friends can be overwhelming as they try to follow the topics of conversations, so they become hermits. A happy medium of social activities and rest contribute to the Quality of Life.

People who suffer with this disease need a balance of sensory stimulation and calming activities. Consider plants or an indoor garden to offer care responsibilities for a person with Alzheimer's. Encourage them to work on a simple project for you; we all need to be needed.

Behavior often has a purpose

Maybe Mom is taking the clothes out of her closet every day. It could be it gives her something to do, she is **bored**, she is "looking" for something which happens more and more or she is so overwhelmed by so MANY clothes she can't decide what to wear! Consider other ideas that could cause her behavior.

New medication could be causing restlessness or anxiety. Ask your pharmacist for the side effects of medication they are taking.

Sadness or depression can contribute to behavior. Sometimes they are frustrated at the things they can't do anymore, sad thinking about what the future may hold, or just a "grey" day when nothing seems quite right.

Too much activity or noise can cause them to be exhausted. Few of us are patient with others when we are tired. Sometimes I think the disease just makes them all want to yell at us with "Don't you understand how tiring it is when everything I see, hear or do is confusing?"

It can be triggered:

It might be something you said, it might be something in the environment, behavior might be due to pain, dehydration, hunger, thirst or exhaustion. Try to keep a written or mental note to consider all these possibilities. Wandering can be caused by boredom (they were looking for something to do), medication side effects and pain from sitting so they began to walk. Be aware if it is the same time of day they become upset. That might suggest it is hunger, thirst, tired or another reason. If we can figure out what might trigger the behavior, we might be able to prevent it.

Sometimes a loved one can become physically aggressive or find a weapon to threaten others. The disease is telling them you are a threat!

If the person becomes violent or aggressive

- Go to a safe place in the house and call for help.

- Remove any weapons from the house (sharp kitchen knives need to be stored in secret place).

- Keep emergency numbers easily accessible.

- Call their doctor for admittance to a "behavioral" unit. Then you can call 911 to take them if necessary and you have DPOA. Even though the behavioral unit sounds scary, this unit often just balances their body chemistry with the drugs they are taking, or tries to discover another reason for their agitated or dangerous behavior. Something you can't do this at home.

Real world is overwhelming

Events in their past often have emotional memory tied to them. It can be sadness, affection, pleasure, anger or nostalgia. But they have lost the ability to attach an emotional feeling to current events. There are many professionals that suggest a person with dementia can't learn new things.

There is no reality in their world and they often can't tell between TV stories and real life! My mom became so upset with the news (she listened to the news most every day of her life before she was ill) that we put the history channel on and she was so excited they "were" currently building the Hoover dam!

They can't tell the difference between truth and a lie. If we tell them their car is in the shop (when it is fine we just don't want them to drive), we call that "therapeutic fibbing". We tell children that there is a Santa Claus, Easter Bunny and Tooth Fairy! Why? Because it improves the quality and fun of their life! It is the same for our loved ones with this disease. We want them safe and enjoying what life they have. Sometimes we don't need all the truth.

People with this disease remember long ago, live in the present and cannot plan for the future. They can't make an emotional connection to a current event to remember.

There is still so much mystery about the symptoms and behaviors (which new research suggests symptoms may not develop until 10-20 years after it has begun to destroy the brain).

Here is example for all of us:

Have you noticed that when you reach a certain age everything is uphill? Groceries are heavier, stairs are steeper, parking lots are bigger and the merchandise in the stores is overwhelming! People are less considerate, they talk in whispers and they don't hold the doors open.

Our reactions.

Sometimes the way we COMMUNICATE affects many of the behaviors of a person with Alzheimer's. **It isn't what we say, but how we say it!**

- Instead of saying "there is no one here but us" try, "I can tell you are worried and frightened, tell me who you think is here?"(If they seem paranoid.)

- Try to be a patient listener, people with dementia become frustrated, restless and agitated sometimes when we don't understand them!

- Use a checklist in your mind- hunger, thirst, tired, bathroom or Pain. Solve the easy answers first.

- Be aware of your body language, tell your name and who you are (don't say "Remember I am…), smile and make eye contact.

- Try to help them remember a SPECIAL time! (Their wedding day, a homerun, First job, etc.) Everyone wants you to appreciate that there is a **PERSON INSIDE THE DISEASE!**

- Behaviors can make the caregivers' life miserable and often the person with dementia would be embarrassed to know they had acted that way. Diseases do awful things to our minds and bodies.

My thoughts:

These are the behaviors that make this disease so difficult. No one talks about the cussing, agitation, violent behavior, urinating all over the house, the yelling or the panic when they have wandered out the door. These are people we love and care for. Every day is different so what calmed them today doesn't work tomorrow. We look at their face and they are the mother we love, and then we look in their eyes, and no one is home. This is an emotional, physical and mental roller coaster! Sometimes nothing works. But many of us have been down this road, and know the feeling. Reach out for help, join support groups, contact the Alzheimer's 24/7 helpline 1-800-272-3900, ask for books, websites, news articles. Turn to friends or those in your church and remember there are 3.5 million others who are currently walking the road too! You are not alone.

CHAPTER 5

Dealing with the diagnosis

Now you know they are sick, you understand some of why their behavior has changed but how do you deal with the changes?

How do you help someone who doesn't want to be helped, because they are fine?

Often in the early stages of the disease the person may be adamant about not wanting your help. They are afraid of losing their "cover" and don't want others to know how bad it is. Sometimes when children, relatives or friends try to help (with cleaning, finances, transportation, etc.) people with Alzheimer's can be mean and nasty to them. Who wants their parent yelling at them like they were 10-years-old again? How long can we turn a blind eye to dents in the car or burned pots and pans? What do we do?

We have a diagnosis, now what?

Fear, sadness, pictures of people in a wheelchair worry, ignorance of the disease, not wanting to be a "burden," and nursing home concerns all come to mind. Shock usually sets in for all involved. The person with Alzheimer's may not remember the diagnosis from the doctor, or may deny it many times in the days to come. It is OK if they don't remember. Being aware they have the disease will probably affect their behavior and/or reasoning skills.

Consider starting a conversation about "**quality of life**" choices. Unfortunately we all die. But someone or a family will be responsible for making choices when your loved one is not able. It feels better to do that if you had these discussions while your loved one can.

Quality of life choices

Where do I want to spend the rest of my life?

Does your loved one want to spend their life near family or in the home they have lived for many years? There are pros and cons to both of those choices. It will be less confusing to stay in the home as it is familiar and they know where the bathroom is and for a while they can drive to local stores. But as the disease progresses, it becomes more of a burden to the spouse or child that lives closest. Change is hard for everyone, but if moving is the decision, the person with Alzheimer's will be able to adjust earlier in the disease when they are more cognitive and may still make friends. Sometimes safety measures and "cleaning out" are easier when they are able to make decisions about what to do. Don't make choices for parents or spouses. TALK ABOUT THE PROS AND CONS of where to live. Remembering that the person with Alzheimer's likely won't recall this conversation. You can always confirm later that you had this discussion. Give them time to consider the options.

Being nearer to grandchildren sometimes makes everyone's' life better. Many parents decline this offer because they don't want to be a "burden." Loving and living with other people we care about is not a BURDEN. It is the price we pay for caring about others. For everyone who TAKES flowers to a person in need, there must be a person in need willing to ACCEPT help. It has to be a two way street.

Often people who have Alzheimer's want to stay close to friends. But immediate family need to consider who will help with behavior problems, hospital stays, doctor visits, or arrange in-home help? Many times long-distance caregivers can manage with visits and phone calls, but eventually as the disease progresses they all need more care.

How do I want to spend the rest of my life?

Does your loved one have a 'bucket list" or dreams yet to be fulfilled?

Did your loved one always want to go to the Grand Canyon? A family cruise? Or write a book? We all have hopes and dreams for the future, but the person with Alzheimer's disease just had a WAKE-UP call, they are sick and they need to enjoy life now!

See if family or friends can make some of those dreams come true if possible. Everyone will feel better for the effort. The time can seem very short between diagnosis and not being able to travel or do the things they love. A hospital stay, pneumonia, flu, or a fall can make the disease progress faster. Sometimes at the beginning of the disease, they don't want to go out and do things because of depression. Later is due to the unfamiliar. Try to support their dreams during this time an encourage them to make those dreams happen.

Family meetings

Have a family meeting. Write down the pros and cons, make a plan for when the living arrangements don't work, be informed about living with someone with Alzheimer's before you offer to have them move in, and lastly, call the Department of Aging in your area and ask about resources that can help them stay in their home, if that is a choice. Only death lasts forever, and life changes our plans. But by being educated about the disease, planning for legal paper work, making sure safety measures are taken and allowing for dreams to come true while they can, everyone should have a better quality of life.

We are all so busy with our lives; no one wants to carve out "extra" time to take care of Mom or Dad, unless we have to. As my mom became more confused, it was hard for her if I wasn't in her room all the time. Unfortunately my mother-in-law became ill and needed my attention. The guilt I felt when she would accuse me of abandoning her to "strangers", was overwhelming.

Heart attacks, hospital stays and surgery all get our attention, but memory loss must be because they are getting old so they shouldn't need our attention. The child that lives closest gets hit with the biggest responsibility and usually first notices when something is wrong. People and couples that have a "secret" of dementia don't want anyone to know, including family.

- Start with communicating with other family members about signs or symptoms.

- Make sure everyone is aware of the 10 warning signs.

- Watch for memory loss, anger and/or agitation, paranoia, bathing difficulties, dressing problems, taking walks and becoming disorientated, and following the caregiver everywhere.

- It is important to let parents have their independence as long as possible, but often by hiding the disease the caregiver or spouse becomes ill.

- The stress, physical, emotional and mental energy it takes to cover and compensate for the person with dementia becomes overwhelming! This disease frequently makes two people sick.

Be prepared

Everyone should have Durable Power of Attorney (DPOA) for health care and financial decisions. If your loved one with Alzheimer's is admitted to the hospital, you will need this paperwork to make decisions for him/her. Sometimes it is easier to start with having a loved one put your name on the HIPPA form doctors require. It doesn't give you power, but allows you and the doctor to exchange information.

If your person with dementia is younger (50 year old to 60 year old) consider choices such as Long Term Care Insurance, what will a diagnosis do to their regular insurance, what about their job? Once there is a diagnosis from a doctor, that information can affect all these things. So have your plans and paper work together.

Write down questions for the doctor. We can't remember all the concerns we have. Be sure they have done blood tests, brain scans, mental tests and have examined family history.

Go with a positive attitude. These are the "wake-up" calls of life. Every day we live we have the chance for bad news or good. As we age, everyone has something wrong with them: migraines, diabetes, allergies, heart disease, cancer, etc. All of these "conditions" could kill you. Yes, the symptoms of Alzheimer's are different. They are sad and much harder to live with. Accepting what life brings is the first step to managing it. You don't have to go down the journey alone, and there is information to give you skills to help.

My thoughts:

It helped me to understand and accept my mom's behavior when I knew the disease was responsible for her actions! At first, I thought it was something I was saying or doing. Maybe there was something else wrong with her, and we needed more doctor visits and tests. Even with her mother and sister having this disease, I couldn't believe, MY MOTHER had it. I blamed it on past illness, medications, age….No one wants to willingly face this journey or road. I was scared, angry, tired, frustrated and felt inadequate. Like many of you, I was busy with a job and children. My fathers' death had left me responsible for all his estate, and now to become a caregiver to my mom left me very overwhelmed.

CHAPTER 6

Daily issues with dementia

Be vigilant

Many doctors ask the right questions, but don't pursue alternative ways to see the problem. For example: the doctor would ask my mom if she was depressed or having trouble remembering? She said NO of course. Depression meant she couldn't "cope" with life and admitting memory problems wasn't going to happen! Elderly people can have some memory problems, so often even Physicians blame it on aging. ALZHEIMER'S IS NOT NORMAL AGING! The answer to the question, "How are you?" is almost always "fine." There is a new National Alzheimer's Plan to help Dementia-Primary Care doctors with this cycle for diagnosis. It involves more screening for patients with warning signs and regular check-ups of the caregiver, also. Family input needs to be mandatory. The person with Alzheimer's doesn't know if they have been eating, and will tell you they have been eating to protect their memory loss!

Use non-confrontational dialogue to get involved in office visits, like" Let me drive you, traffic is bad today" or "Why don't I take notes, in case you have questions later?" because part of the short term memory problem means they don't remember what the doctor told them!

Many families told of going to several doctors to get a diagnosis, because the one their family used for years didn't do appropriate tests despite the family's list of symptoms. Sometimes doctors think families are too emotional and don't share important information.

People with Alzheimer's disease are vulnerable

Go to banks and places where their money is kept; talk with the manager about your loved one's disease (spread awareness). If you have a DPOA for financial, make a copy for them and ask them to call if there are large withdrawals from your loved one's accounts.

Talk with Lawyers about the best way to protect your loved one from abuse. This includes family that will ask for money, knowing your loved one will forget they have given them some and give more. Telemarketers and charities may also be a hazard because your loved one may donate several times daily, not remembering they just sent a check the day before!

We must learn to talk with our loved ones suffering from Alzheimer's in a new way. Their brain does not process information the same.

People with a form of dementia, can use "salad" words. It means they mix up real words, so they don't make any sense! Some days they may use just verbs or just nouns. But usually they are just struggling to "find" words. We can't change THEIR communication skills but we can change ours!

My mom kept saying "shoes" one day, so we guessed, where the shoes were, different shoes, new shoelaces to find out what she needed. Turns out her shoes hurt and she wanted new ones. Some days, twenty questions works to find an answer!

1. Communication

It isn't WHAT you say to them, it is HOW you say it! That is a rule we use in our lives every day but in a different way. We tell children to believe in the Tooth Fairy. Is it lying? With a person who has Alzheimer's, we call it "therapeutic fibbing." It means we don't always need the whole truth. It's like emphasizing the positive. Often because of the disease, they can't process cause and effect, no matter how much we explain. So we say things that we hope will improve the quality of their lives instead. Do children need an Easter Bunny, Santa Claus and Tooth Fairy? No, but sure makes life a lot more fun for us all!

Talking to a person with Alzheimer's is like that. If they don't remember all the details the doctor said about the disease, do you need to repeat it? Sometimes it is kinder to say they have a disease that affects their memory and you both will deal with it one day at a time, because their brain may not be able to process it all. Do people with Alzheimer's know that their behavior has anything to do with the disease? Usually not. Here are some examples with ideas for a response:

- When you are concerned about their housekeeping, try "Mom, some days I'm really tired of house cleaning, would you come help me clean out some closets and then I will come help you clean?" Instead of, "Mom, you have too much junk in your closet to find anything!" (Remember people with Alzheimer's can become hoarders because they can't make decisions.)

- If you notice pills are still in their box and obviously not being taken, you can suggest an automatic pill box to make life easier. Tell them you hate filling your own boxes of pills could you help?

- **Validate their feelings**

  We all need to feel valuable and that what we think is important. If your loved one becomes angry or frustrated try "I can tell you are really angry about that... sounds like they weren't listening to how you feel. Verify what you think they said by rephrasing or repeating.

- **Redirect their thoughts.**

  Offer them something to eat or drink while they tell you the problem. (Many times people with Alzheimer's are hungry or thirsty and can't remember where to get food or water, so they can become angry.)Focus on positive experiences. Remind them everything is OK.

- **Reminisce about a happy memory-**

  We all want to spend our lives remembering the "good times," happy things and time we spent with others that we laughed! Often these memories help us relax and dwell on good things, instead of what we are really angry about. Everyone needs a friend or family to listen to their problems, but people with Alzheimer's lose the ability to reach out.

  Often grandchildren and sometimes children don't want to visit their loved one because they don't know what to say. There is a magazine called Reminisce (www.reminisce.com) that has pictures from the 40's, 50's, and 60's that reminds us of happy times. There may be a picture of a '60 Chevy that was their first car! Use these pictures to ask questions. How did you buy your first car? What was your first car? How did you learn to cook? Did you have a prom dress like that?

There are books called "For my grandchildren" that have questions about "Who was president when you were a child", "How did you meet Grandma?" "What is your favorite color"? These are good activities to do with people who have the disease. It gives them something to do that they know, and it gives family a record of their past, what did they do, what made them happy, what are their best memories? (You may need some of these memories to divert their attention if behavior becomes a problem!) Before they die people want to know they have made a difference, remind them of their accomplishments! It improves the quality of their life.

- **Always speak to them as an adult-**

Use a low pitch, calm tone. Address them by their name. Try to listen for their emotional message. Watch for smiles (reinforce those), fear of the future, sadness, or anger (could be at another family member, staff, or spouse.) Reflect what you see or hear, but never say "Don't be sad." We all feel sad some times. Remind them you are there to help and get through it together! Never speak about them in front of them. A person with dementia usually understands more than we think.

Sometimes they are angry about everything! Nothing you say works. The medications that are given for this disease are to slow the progression of the disease and help with daily living, they cannot bring back memory. Part of the reason to get a proper diagnosis is for medication to deal with anger, hallucinations, paranoia or agitation. They may not alter the symptoms of the disease, but changing medication, such as antidepressants, anti-anxiety drugs, or anti psychotics can help with behavior, when all else fails.

Your loved one could be afraid of getting older or what lies ahead, restless (anxiety can make it hard to sit still), frustrated that it is harder to do the things they used to do, sleepless because some of the medication and even paranoid because they don't want anyone to notice they are forgetting. These things can all cause behaviors problems.

Use these communication tips:

- Be aware of your body language, it may say more than words.

- Be conscious of the environment, is it dark in their room?

- Identify yourself, SMILE!

- Speak slowly, calmly and use simple words, wait for a response.

- Turn down the TV or other distracting noise so they can focus.

- Phrase questions so the answer is "yes" or "no".

- It is Ok to laugh, they will laugh with you.

- Sometimes touching is reassuring.

- Always speak to them like an adult.

- Sometimes gestures or pictures help.

- Be aware of THEIR facial expressions, to show pain, pleasure, etc.

- Never argue, disagree, embarrass or correct what they say.

- Don't talk about them like they aren't there.

- Create opportunities to laugh or smile.

- Singing sometimes relaxes everyone.

2. Eliminate easy causes

You have tried talking to them in a different way and they are still upset mad or restless, what else can you do?

Start with the obvious things: sight, hearing, medication and/or pain problems. Could their behavior be caused from one of these things? People with Alzheimer's can go to the eye doctor (because "There must be something wrong with my glasses.") when unfortunately, their vision is usually fine but their MIND can't process what they see anymore!

The same applies to hearing problems. Sometimes hearing aids get lost, need new batteries or just as with sight issues, they can't process what they hear!

Side effects of medication can also make a person act differently. A person with Alzheimer's can't problem solve to consider if the medication isn't working, (sometimes it can take weeks for medication to kick in) the side effects are making them sick or they need a different kind of medication.

Pain makes everyone grumpy! My favorite story is of a lady who had back trouble and had taken Lortab most of the last few years of her life due to pain. But the family member called to say she wasn't taking it anymore since she had been diagnosed with Alzheimer's. Do you think because she has Alzheimer's she doesn't have pain? Usually it is the same problem as seeing and hearing, **they can't process pain!** Investigate to see if some pain reliever helps with behavior. There were some studies done about comparing pain with an Alzheimer's patient needing hip surgery and someone just needing hip surgery. The people without Alzheimer's need up to three times more pain reliever for the same surgery. This is most likely because they were able to process their pain and ask for pain relievers accordingly.

Sometimes people with Alzheimer's don't want to get up in the morning. Many of us, as we age have arthritis and are stiff in the morning, so we stretch or take anti-inflammatory medications. A person with this disease can't think of ways to help with the pain.

To deal with these issues consider aromatherapy. Studies have shown that the scent of lavender can be calming and help with sleep. There are room sprays, body lotion and scents that plug into the wall. Also be sure that your loved one is getting enough sunlight. Many people with dementia suffer from a lack of Vitamin D, Seasonal affective Disorder (SAD).

3. Exhaustion!

Try to imagine what it must be like to lose a little of your mind every day, to work diligently to keep your independence, and with every conversation you must be "on guard" so your memory problems don't show. That might change your behavior too!

Families either shy away or take charge to move their loved one. But life is just baby steps. We don't expect children to talk in sentences right away. It takes everyone a while to accept, learn and adjust to any type of disease!

Offer people with Alzheimer's acceptable choices, without telling them what to do. Suggest ideas, make them think it was THEIR idea, and begin with a plan. Only you need to remember the plan. Tell them "You and I talked about this, and agreed it was a good idea." Always remember **"Do the choices I make for my loved one with Alzheimer's improve the quality of their life?"**

4. How you can help them

Before you actually become their caregiver or move them into your home, be aware of the repercussions. Can your marriage survive you being on call 24/7, sleepless nights, no privacy, emotional turmoil that comes from caring for someone you love and the effect on children and grandchildren?

Rarely do all siblings share the responsibility equally. Some will never admit that their family member has Alzheimer's, others say they live too far to help, some say they are just too busy with their own family and lives to help. SOMEONE HAS TO HELP!

Sometimes we choose to be a Caregiver, and sometimes it is chosen for us. Either way, just like life, there are rewards along the way!

My thoughts:

Unfortunately Alzheimer's disease is not like any other disease. Just making sure they are safe and eating is not enough. Because of the nature of it, there is usually anger, depression, confusion, disorientation. These symptoms can make others around them miserable too. This disease strikes randomly. Physical illness like a stroke, flu, pneumonia can make them suddenly worse.

CHAPTER 7

Ideas for dealing with the symptoms

Here are some ideas for the symptoms families deal with:

- **Memory loss**

   Families say it is so hard because they keep repeating the same things over and over. Yes, it is often like a record going around and around. Sometimes we can divert them when they start the same story with a walk outside, a snack, a good memory from the past, or ask for their help or advice about something. (We all like to be needed!)

   Be aware of memory loss that affects their daily living; remembering to take their pills, forgetting keys, using the appliances, getting lost while driving, forgetting how to make a meal. These things can affect their safety and wellbeing. It is OK to have momentary lapses about working the microwave, but if it happens often, it can interfere with their ability to eat or their general safety.

- **Shadowing**

   People who suffer from dementia can follow their caregivers from room to room, ask questions repeatedly, ask when the caregiver is coming home and where they are going, become needy about everything, and lose skills they have been doing forever! We call this Shadowing.

Even time alone in the shower is compromised by the presence of a mate with dementia. The caregiver becomes the eyes, (as depth perception and reading become difficult) the ears, (as processing what they hear is harder) the provider, (they fix the food and know where it is) and the "keeper of time" (people with Dementia lose a sense of time, they don't know when it is time to eat or go to bed.)

It is exhausting to those around them. Their spouse, caregiver or family member becomes their brain. They depend on the other person to eat, to sleep, to find the bathroom, etc. Often they only feel safe in their presence. They literally become someone else's shadow!

The person with Alzheimer's begins to feel rejected when the caregiver tries to withdraw from them. This can lead to negative behavior such as shouting, hitting, or biting.

Comfort them with words of reassurance and love. Put duct tape on the floor to help them find the bathroom on their own, or distract them with tasks such as sorting the socks. Repeat with love: YOU ARE SAFE, I LOVE YOU, and EVERYTHING WILL BE OK! If you need a bathroom break to be alone for a few minutes, try setting a timer they can see and hear, tell them you will be back before it goes off, and then give them a task to work on. This is a stage of the disease and will be replaced with other behavior. Be patient, and try to remember we all need each other, sometime, somewhere or somehow.

- **Anger and agitation**

  It is very difficult to deal with or be with people who are angry at everyone. Sometimes it is triggered by fear of losing control of their life or fear that family will start telling them what to do. They don't know that eventually the disease will take control.

  Just because we understand why they are angry, we also need to know how to deal with it every day. For example, my mom used to be angry at the news and afraid, every time she heard of a violent crime somewhere. It is the everyday triggers that you must learn to deal with.

Here are some ideas for dealing with anger and agitation:

- **Reduce caffeine, watch for sugar overload.**

- **Simplify their life.**

- **Structure is helpful; routine helps them balance the familiar.**

- **Pictures of family (with names attached) can offer a sense of security.**

- **Soft music instead of "fast moving" TV can be calming.**

- **Guns and sharp knives should be put away!**

- Support independence as long as they are safe.

- Acknowledge their frustrations and anger.

- Distract with food or drink.

- Call 911 if they are a danger to themselves or others!

If you are afraid they will harm you or others, be prepared to:

Call their doctor and describe their behavior and ask if you can have them admitted to a behavior unit at a hospital. Will your loved one be angry at you? Yes, but they are very angry now, that is why you called 911. Usually because of the nature of their short- term memory problems, they don't remember you called.

Leave the house and call from neighbors' if you feel physically threatened.

- **Paranoia**

This symptom can often occur early in the disease. It means that there is damage to the part of the brain that helps us decide what is real and what isn't. They can become jealous of a spouse they have been married to for years. Even seeing themselves in a mirror may be scary because they don't remember what they look like and could be afraid of the person in the mirror. Their paranoia or hallucinations are VERY real to them. It can be just part of Alzheimer's.

Encourage their spouse to be more affectionate or use loving words to help if suspicious. Help them to look for things that they think are stolen. (It might help to have a 2nd purse with vital information like social security card, that is kept in a safe place by caregiver, in case they lose or hide the current one).Make sure there is enough light in the room so they can better find things.

My mom used to call and be angry that we had taken all her money and she couldn't find any cash in her purse or drawers. So we gave her $40, showed it to her and told her to put where she wanted.

Of course no matter where she put it, she couldn't find it. In her confused state, if she couldn't find it, "someone must have stolen it". Don't take these accusations personally; it is all part of the disease! The good news is she found and lost that money many times in 2 years.

Be aware that people that suffer from Alzheimer's have been known to go to the bank and withdraw money, only to later not remember what happened to it. Then come home and they may then blame someone else for the withdrawal.

• **Hallucinations**

This can be caused by side effects of medication or the disease affecting their brain, which can keep them from processing common occurrences. For example: the air conditioner causes the curtain to blow and move, but a person with Alzheimer's may think it is an intruder! This story illustrates how a person with Alzheimer's may process something simple, such as passing by a mirror:

An old lady has moved into my house. She usually keeps out of sight, but when I pass a mirror, there she is obliterating my gorgeous face and body. I think she is stealing money from me, I go to the ATM and withdraw $100.00 and a few days later it is gone. I don't spend money that fast. My food is disappearing at an alarming rate, good stuff like candy, cookies and ice cream. I'm sure she is tampering with my scale! She messes with my papers and files until I can't find anything!

- **Sundowning and sleeplessness**

  Sometimes even in the early stages of the disease, they can have nightmares and not sleep well. One of the side effects of a common Alzheimer's drug, Aricept, is nightmares. Namenda, another common Alzheimer's drug, can cause extreme hallucinations. We all know how tired and sometimes irritable we are if we don't sleep well. Start with easy choices, could it be medication, arthritis pain, caffeine, too much light, incontinence, or just not tired due to lack of activity? Not sleeping well can affect everyone.

  Sundowning is very common with this disease but isn't usually recognized as a symptom of the disease. It usually happens late in the day or early evening. Sundowning means a restless, pacing, agitated, or even wandering in or out of the house when the sun goes down. It is sometimes caused by shadows that are scary, the coming darkness, exhaustion, pain because they have been sitting all afternoon and now are stiff, confusion with night/day as days get shorter and their biological clock is trying to change, they get cold as darkness comes, or they wake up from a nap and are disoriented. All these factors may cause or contribute to this symptom. It may start in the late afternoon and last into the evening.

Things to help deal with Sundowning:

- Increase activity during the day.

- Offer food or drink to help them "wake" after resting.

- Plan bigger meals for lunch so they will have their spouse's attention during dinner preparation, when the sun goes down.

- Think of activities for late afternoon or early evening to help them ignore environmental changes in the day.

- Turn on lights before dusk.

- Be aware of staircases, depth perception may make them dangerous.

- Maybe offer pain relief medication.

- Make sure poisons are in a safe place. (They may not remember what it is).

Bathing

We all have been bathing ourselves since we were children. How can bathing possibly be a problem?

People with Alzheimer's often have trouble with bathing and hygiene. Sometimes we begin to notice with body odor or spots on everything they wear. Can you imagine a tactful way to ask your mom when she had a shower last? If a suggestion is made, often the person with Alzheimer's becomes angry, indignant, appalled, or defensive!

Sometimes they forget to bathe because they think they have already bathed, they don't remember WHY you need to bathe, it is painful to bathe because their skin is so sensitive and thin or it is exhausting to figure out the shower and go through the process. Depression can contribute to lack of interest in bathing, as well.

We all are motivated by something! We get up and go to work because we get a paycheck, we clean the house because it looks better and hopefully reduce germs and we help others because it feels good! To encourage a person to bathe, we try to motivate. "I have a new scented body wash, I want you to try," "Why don't you go ahead and shower and the cookies will be out of the oven by then," or "I have some new music that sounds great in the bathroom." Always offer choices, "Do you want to take a bath or shower?"

- To help with bathing/hygiene also try: Adopt their bathing routine, as much as possible. (Suggest a shower in the morning if that was their pattern or that salon always washed her hair.)

- Encourage them to wash all over because their skin is so dry and it might feel better with this new moisturizing soap.

- Always respect their modesty with towels.

- Make sure the bathroom and water are warm enough.

- Check the lighting so they can see what they are doing.

- Be aware of needed grab-bars, and always use a colored bath mat in the tub (it helps with depth perception for them to get into tub). Don't encourage people who have Alzheimer's, to sit in the bathtub as they forget how to lift themselves and get out. It is hard for others to help as they are wet! Often a shower-stool or chair is helpful. A hand held showerhead is also a good idea, as it gives the person more control.

- Never leave them alone, always be nearby to help.

- Consider a" towel bath" for a soothing alternative and to break the struggle with bathing. The towel bath uses a large bath towel and washcloths dampened in a plastic bag of warm water and no-rinse soap. Large bath-blankets are used to keep the person covered, dry and warm while the warm washcloths are massaged over the body. (See website at the end of book for details, "Bathing without a Battle".)

- Use a different word for bath or shower such as "Let's go freshen-up in the bathroom" or "Dad, let me see how your shower head is working, let's go in the bathroom and look."

- Consider some pain reliever before the bath, to help with skin sensitivity.

Dressing

This daily activity may become more of an issue as it is hard for them to decide about clothes in the closet (when there are many choices) and so they wear the same thing, every day! Sometimes early in the disease easy decisions are difficult. My mom couldn't decide what to have on a menu, so she always had whatever I was having! She was always dressed smartly, but began to wear the same soiled clothes everyday as the disease progressed.

People suffering from Alzheimer's may become overwhelmed, uncooperative and resistant to activities of daily living. Every day we make hundreds of easy decisions. But as the confusion grows, these decisions make them feel out of control, frustrated, afraid of making the wrong choice, rushed and exhausted!

- Simplify their closets: Make sure everything goes together.

  Sometimes get two of the same outfit, so you can wash one.

  Eliminate too many buttons, difficult zippers or shirts that are too tight over their head. Sometimes their attention span becomes too short for the task at hand. Keep encouraging and let them sit and rest if necessary. Respect their privacy with blinds closed and doors shut. As the disease progresses, there may be a need for laying the clothes on a dark bedspread in the order needed.

Driving

Unfortunately driving is life threatening for everyone, the person with Alzheimer's and everyone else on the road. It is difficult to decide when a person with Alzheimer's should stop driving and still respect their independence! All persons with Alzheimer's will eventually become unable to drive, because of the nature of the disease.

Driving represents freedom, independence, and ability. Try to imagine your world if you couldn't drive, how would you feel? Alzheimer's is unpredictable. Just because yesterday they could drive to the store without getting lost or in an accident, doesn't mean they can today.

Often times it is easier for spouses and family members to turn a blind eye to driving problems. No one wants to offend or agitate the person with Alzheimer's about a very sensitive issue. Recently there was a man 53 years old who had dementia, was driving the wrong way and hit and killed a pregnant woman and her husband. Now the courts must decide who is to blame. Did the family know he had dementia and turned a blind eye to his driving, should the doctor who made the diagnosis done more, or is no one to blame because he had dementia?

Consider this:

- Find a balance. One fender bender does not mean it is time to take the keys. But many dents in the car may be a bigger problem.

- Ask yourself if you would let your grandchild ride in the car with them, or you would cross the street in front of them?

- Watch for warning signs like: riding the brake, incorrect signaling, increased agitation while driving, driving at inappropriate speeds, or delayed response to unexpected situations.

- Make an alternate transportation plan. Start with friends or family who could pick them up. Tell them you just want a chance to visit!

- Share concerns about driving with their doctor, sometimes driving issues are better addressed by a person of authority.

- If taxi or bus transportation is an option, write down the details or make arrangements for them. Tell them they are worth it!

- Check for other resources from aging programs for transportation.

- Consider home deliveries for medicine or groceries.

- See if a family member can take turns helping with errands for a day.

So how do you have that conversation about not driving?

Before you have a conversation about driving, make sure the person with Alzheimer's is not thirsty, hungry or exhausted, as this could make them easily agitated or upset. Approach your loved one with only a couple of family members so they don't feel ganged up on.

Conversation could start with, "the doctor said there were some changes in your medication that could affect your driving, " or, "You always said it was better to be safe than sorry, and we are concerned about your driving with this disease."

The Alzheimer's Association has great material to help families with this driving discussion be sure to ask about the Hartford Insurance Driving handbook.

Wandering

People with Alzheimer's can wander from their home suddenly. They can come to a busy street and forget how to cross or just walk down the street to a neighbor.

Wandering can be very dangerous, especially if there are extreme temperatures in the weather. Due to depth perception problems, the risk for falling also becomes high in an unfamiliar environment. Wandering can occur on foot or in a car. Sometimes they wander because they are looking for something familiar.

To help prevent Wandering:

- Put a stop sign on back of the front door.

- Try a black mat in front of the door, they sometimes think it is a hole and won't cross it.

- Put a chime over the door, so you will know if they have opened the door. You may need locks up high they can't reach for security reasons.

- Provide appropriate exercise. (Walk at the mall, in the garden or museum.)

- Remove hats, coats, scarves, or other things that may trigger a need to go out.

- Consider a GPS watch or shoes, just in case.

- Night lights often provide comfort in the dark.

- Have a current picture of your loved one, to provide identification to police, neighbors, etc. in case your loved one wanders out.

- Think about a Medic-alert bracelet for identification and medical needs.

- Use a jacket with reflective tape.

Often people with Alzheimer's have what is called an Unsteady Gait. This means their balance and depth perception affect their walking. This increases the chance for falling and makes wandering even more dangerous. Families describe it as "they shuffle" their feet. My Mom did this because she couldn't perceive where to put her foot down. She would edge her foot over the curb and down to the street level. Patterns on rugs can make it harder to tell the floor. Medicare used to pay for physical therapy for Alzheimer's people. It can help their balance some.

Wanting to go home

Many times people who suffer with this disease say they "Just want to go home." Most times it isn't the home they usually live in, but often it is a childhood home. Unfortunately, taking them to a childhood home doesn't help, as it is a memory in their brain. Home may mean a time when they were well and normal. They may say this if they are at a restaurant, friends, store, or an activity center. Unfortunately taking them home to their residence doesn't always solve the problem.

Tips to try:

- Go for a ride or walk. Sometimes on returning, their home looks familiar.

- Use validation to reflect how they are feeling and remind them they are safe.

- Make note of the time of day this agitation occurs. Maybe plan an activity, like a snack for that time of day.

- Try to redirect with reminiscing.

All people with Alzheimer's don't wander. But we all have days when we want to "get away from it all!" Sometimes that is a bath, a trip or just a movie.

Remember this is a progressive disease, and different for everyone but for most people as the brain begins to degenerate, activity is more difficult.

Activities

So we have left a person with Alzheimer's alone at home all day, while we all have gone about our tasks for the day! Remember that for a person with Alzheimer's, finishing tasks becomes difficult for them, finding things can be an all-day task, initiative to do hobbies they love is nonexistent, and tracking is very hard. Try leaving some tasks for them to do in an obvious place. Have them sort and match socks. (Someone has to do it!) Other household chores, like vacuuming, could be helpful to everyone. Keeping busy with activities can help with problems in behavior and emotional issues such as loneliness.

Other tips to try:

- Encourage a friend to stop for coffee.

- Be cautious about TV shows that could cause hallucinations, aggression, or paranoia. Instead, try something like Funniest Home Videos.

- If there is safety issues with leaving them home alone consider having them volunteer at a day care center or senior center.

- Check out books and hand-outs about activities from the Alzheimer's association.

Sometimes if you can afford it, consider a companion to listen to their stories of the past over and over.

- Let them do as much as they can as long as they can, safely!

My thoughts:

Not everyone with Alzheimer's will have all these symptoms. But by knowing about them you can be prepared. Your loved one is not intentionally being obstinate, annoying, wearing dirty clothes, or getting your attention by being lost.

CHAPTER 8

The problems of daily living

Be informed

Learn all you can about Alzheimer's and types of dementia. The Alzheimer's Association has lots of information, the internet, ask your doctor, talk to friends who have been down this journey; check out books. Ignorance is rarely bliss.

Medication

Most doctors will put your loved one on medication after diagnosis. But it may or may not help with any of the symptoms. As the disease progresses you may need other medication to help with depression, anger or sleeping.

- Keep records. Your loved one may not remember why they need this medication. When did they start this medication? (Medications take time to get into the system and work. Could be 24 hours or 3 weeks, ask pharmacist.) It doesn't help until it has had time to work in their system

- What are the side effects? (Ask a pharmacist for most common.)

- What type of medication is it? - Alzheimer's medication, antidepressant, anti-anxiety, antibiotic?

- What is it for? The two most common Alzheimer's drugs are to slow the progression of the disease and help with daily living. None help with memory loss.

- How often do they take it? Make sure you have a pillbox that provides different times of day if needed.

- Who is going to help them remember to take it? - Short term memory loss is an early symptom. Sometimes they think it has been a long day, and take the next day's pills!

Often people in the early stages suffer from depression. Before our improved diagnosis testing it was thought Alzheimer's was only a type of depression. Sometimes people become depressed after they receive a diagnosis. Others say it isn't that bad they only have dementia! Because they were unaware that depression can be a symptom of dementia.

Watch for withdrawal such as not wanting to go out to restaurants or making excuses to friends about not meeting them for lunch. (I knew a lady in early stages of the disease that missed her granddaughter's wedding because she was too depressed to come out of her room!) Some are concerned that the 2 drugs usually prescribed for dementia don't seem to help. But often anti-depressant, anxiety, or anti-psychotic drugs are needed instead to control the symptoms of disease; which hopefully, improves the quality of life for the caregiver and the person with dementia.

Depression

It is important not to have anyone take too much medication, because even aspirin has side effects. But the clock is ticking for us all, and anything that will improve the quality of life for the time we have, is often a good idea. It doesn't mean that people with Alzheimer's will have to take antidepressants forever. Usually it is just a stage of the disease when depression is worse. This could be the early part when they are afraid of what lies ahead with this disease, they feel helpless against it. Often the doctor asks the patient if they are depressed. But usually people who are older equate "depressed" with "weak," "unstable" or" lazy," and they do not want to admit they may be depressed.

Many people think once they are on some sort of medicine it will cure it, the troubling symptoms will go away, or they will be fine now. But even if they had cancer, after taking them to treatments and life will not be ever normal. People do recover from cancer, but their lives are rarely normal again. People with Alzheimer's have good days, hours, or weeks, but their brains will never be normal again.

Weight loss or gain

Sometimes people gain weight because they forget they have eaten, so they eat again or can't find anything else to do. Frequently, people with a form of dementia, have an increasing taste for sweet things. This may be due the taste buds that are still sending messages to the brain.

The taste of sweet things is usually the last to go. This can explain weight gain for some people.

Weight loss can be due to medications, they forget how to cook, where to find the food or how to use microwave or stove. Side effects of medication, fatigue and depression can affect appetite.

Eating

Here are some tips that might help stabilize weight:

- Try putting some casseroles in the freezer with detailed instructions about how to cook, temperature and time. Making a note on the cabinet to remind them it is there, may also help.

- Consider placing a note on the dishwasher about where the soap goes and "start" button. (If they ask why it is there, tell them.)

- Look in the refrigerator for expired or spoiled food.

- Offer to go to the grocery store once in a while. How overwhelming most of our supermarkets have become! It may not be worth it for them to go and deal with the confusion of all the products. Suggest a smaller local grocery store, if they insist on going themselves.

- Make yourself aware of any foods your loved one cannot take with his/her medication.

- Make sure they have some of their favorite foods.

- Make a fun note on the cabinet that says, "What yummy thing did you have for lunch or dinner"? (This is important for people living alone. They usually can't tell you what or if they had lunch. My Mom used to say "Oh the usual...")

- Be prepared for changes in food preferences.

- Put water bottles many places to remind them to drink water. Older people aren't used to drinking water and some younger people only drink coffee or pop. Make sure glasses are easy to handle and not too big for their hands. Dehydration has bad repercussions for us all!

- Sometimes eating on a dark colored plate helps us see the food.

Safety and wandering

Even with children we talk about fire drills, calling 911 and crossing the street. These are not children. But making our homes safe is important.

1. Sometimes dementia people in the early stages just need help changing the smoke detector batteries.

2. Everyone needs a fire extinguisher that works, but adding simple directions for use that isn't in small print helps with confusion and age related eyesight.

3. Isn't it more fun to clean out our closets if we have a friend, and maybe cheesecake and coffee for reward? Prevent clutter, and watch for signs of hoarding. Dementia people often let papers, magazines, and clothes accumulate until walking in their house is dangerous. They lose the ability to make decisions about what to keep and are overwhelmed. It's exhausting to clean out closets and sort through papers! Dressing is a problem because there are TOO many choices in their closet!

4. What about a workshop with power tools that could be dangerous, and broken? Accidents happen everywhere, even if our cognitive skills are good. If they have a workshop, go visit with them while they are working one day to be sure they have the ability to work with electrical tools.

5. Some people with Alzheimer's wander. The difference between taking a walk every day and wandering is they can't find their way home and forget traffic rules! This behavior associated with this disease is deadly! There are stories of people wandering onto a golf course and freezing to death or caregivers following their loved one in the car to make them come home, only to have the person who is confused fall from heat exhaustion before they could get them to come home! Preventing wandering is a safety issue. Consider bells or electronic devices on the doors, so other family members will know someone has gone out.

What can you do to make things safe? Here are some things to think about:

- Inspect smoke detectors, hand rails and make sure steps are secure.

- Offer to help with clutter that might make walking hazardous.

- Check driving skills and ride with them. Make sure there is emergency information in the car.

- Extra keys- Can they lock themselves out? Is the security system too confusing? Losing car keys?

- Position locks higher on the door to discourage wandering.

- Consider a stop sign on the back of the door if wandering is an issue.

- There are special devices, such as shoes, that contain a GPS device in them. You may wish to consider some of these products if wandering is an issue for your loved one.

- Store a hat and coat in a safe place, some people won't go out without their favorite hat.

- Tell neighbors that your loved one has a disease so they can be your eyes and ears

- Keep a current photo for identification if you need one.

- Consider an ID bracelet such as the Alzheimer's Association Medic-Alert bracelet.

- Be aware of throw rugs and things on the floor that might be a tripping hazard.

- Be very cautious with stairs. Deteriorating depth perception makes stairs harder to navigate!

- Try duct tape on the stairs for visibility, or consider not going downstairs.

- Be sure hand rails are available.

- Lighting is important!

- Dimming lights at night can help dementia people be aware of the time of day.

- Post large print directions next to the thermostat.

- Sometimes a red dot on a microwave can help highlight the start button or stop button.

- Post emergency phone numbers for family, police and fire in large numbers. Physician's phone numbers should be in a prominent place also.

Lethargy

Sometimes people with dementia don't want to get out of bed because they are in pain, drug side effects from the night before are still making them groggy, they had nightmares from drugs, they are disorientated and don't know where they are, or depression can cause apathy.

Here are some ideas:

- Ask their doctor about some pain medication, give it time to work and try again. As we age, arthritis or activity from the day before can make us stiff in the morning.

- Ask if medication that is making them groggy may be split in the morning and half in the evening.

- Nightmares or vivid dreams can contribute to disorientation. Give them water and have them sit on their bed to get their bearings.

- Sometimes it is OK to be tired. It takes a lot of energy to pretend you aren't confused!

Boredom

"They sit and watch Television all day." As a person becomes more confused it is harder for them to distinguish reality from what they see on TV. My mother became VERY upset watching the news about war, violence, murder, and the state of the world. We all think it is pretty scary. But she would worry about it. Dementia people then watch a CSI or even a Western, and don't realize it is just a story. Sometimes the Weather Channel and nature shows were relaxing.

As their minds struggle to remember, it is difficult to think of other things, besides TV, to do! Sometimes hobbies like knitting, sewing, or reading can take a lot of effort. They forget they used to do that, their minds can't process words to read, or the disease can make them too restless or anxious to sit still.

Studies say that exercise helps give us more energy. Sometimes if we can get a person with dementia involved in exercise, they enjoy it once they get started. Exercise also helps keep them stronger to compensate for balance issues.

Sunshine and fresh air makes us all feel better, if only for a few minutes. Give them a project to work on for you; cutting coupons, folding clothes, arranging silk flowers, break up fresh beans, sort coins to go in wrappers, cut up paper and staple together for scrap paper, polish silver, etc.

My thoughts:

Every family has a different road. Did you know a fastidious dresser can refuse to bathe until the smell drives everyone crazy? Did you know a woman with dementia can become so aggressive she is physically hurting her spouse? Dementia people can also be sexually inappropriate with dress, words and actions. They may expose themselves in public. Bathroom behavior, such as urination, may happen in closets, potted plants or on the carpet in the corner. Some wander until they are cold or lost, and freeze to death. Paranoia can become so severe they won't let anyone in the house help them. People with dementia who find a gun have shot their caregiver. One caregiver woke up with a big knife under the mattress. It is more than memory loss!

CHAPTER 9

Caregivers

Most of us are caregivers in some way. We care for our children, spouses, sick friends, neighbors, co-workers and family young and old. There are lots of names for what we do, but helping someone else is part of life. Do we get mad at our spouse when they don't help, are we angry at a boss who expects the impossible, are we too busy to make soup for a friend who is inconveniently sick, or are we frustrated to take time from our busy lives to help a parent who really doesn't want our help? Yes! **They say at some time in our life we either ARE a caregiver, HAVE BEEN a caregiver or will NEED a caregiver!**

There is a fine line between leaving a confused loved one alone for hours or deciding they might need someone to keep them company and be sure they are safe. Caregivers need time away, but can you really trust them home alone?

Becoming a caregiver who provides ALL these things 24/7 is overwhelming! Spouses have learned to be independent of each other, with their own interests and activities. Parents strive to be independent without the help or intervention of their adult children. Sometimes different interests keep a marriage together, and definitely busy parents may not need their adult children. But age, disease, and time take their toll. Often, we become resentful of a spouse who needs most of our time or a parent who suddenly needs help when we are busy raising a young family with a job of our own.

People with dementia want to be as independent as long as they can. They don't choose to be needy or to have this devastating disease! Sometimes they will even be <u>mean</u> to a caregiver to protect their independence! Remember just because they seem fine and able, doesn't mean they are! We all want to assume they can still cook, bathe, take their pills, and pay their bills. But once it becomes evident that they can't perform these tasks, we have to sacrifice our time, money and energy to help.

Rarely is sickness, death or accidents convenient. There are no second chances, we don't get to go back in time again and decide next time I will help. Waiting to help someone else can be a life or death choice, or it can make a huge difference in the quality of someone's life today.

Some people become caregivers of parents out of guilt, no one else would, or they live the closest. Spouses of people with Alzheimer's have usually made the choice to be a caregiver, but some divorce and leave.

Choose to reach out and help someone, be a CARE-GIVER or CAREPARTNER. People that are caregivers get an opportunity to make memories with the person with Alzheimer's and a chance to laugh and smile with them.

Request from a person with Alzheimer's - (author unknown)

Be patient with me. My brain disease is beyond my control.

Accept me the way I am. I still have something to offer you.

Talk with me and listen to me. I can't always answer, but I do understand the tone of your voice and your expressions of interest.

Because I cannot remember does not mean I am dumb

Be kind to me. Your kindness may be the highlight of my day.

Don't hurry me. Each day I struggle to keep up and understand.

Consider my feelings. I am sensitive to shame, embarrassment, fear, failure, and uncertainty. Don't ignore me.

Treat me with dignity. I am no less of a person because I have Alzheimer's disease. I would do the same for you if our positions were reversed.

Remember my past. Remind me of my previous successes, values and worth.

Remember my present. I am frightened but still a loving member of a family. Break down activities into steps I can handle. I respond to praise and encouragement.

Remember my future. I need hope for tomorrow.

Love me. And your gifts of love will be a blessing of light for all our lives.

Lessons

- If you don't take care of yourself, you can't take care of anyone else! Get your physical, take your medicine, try to rest, check on relief care, have someone to talk with, and PLAN.

- Denial hurts everyone.

- One person can't do everything.

- If the roles were reversed, what would you want them to do for you?

- Have these important conversations about life and death, before it is too late.

- Safety in your home is vital for everyone living there.

- Change isn't easy if you are sick or not.

- People and making memories is more important than things.

- Because Alzheimer's is a slow progressive disease, it gives families and spouses time to plan, learn and prepare for what may lie ahead.

- Be informed and educated. Realize that you are not alone. Ask for help. Information is empowering!

- Accept what you can and cannot change.

- Don't make promises. ("I won't put you in a nursing home" instead say "I will make choices to give you the best quality of life.")

- Use respite care regularly. Avoid being a martyr. This is your life, too.

- Laughter is truly the best medicine.

- Be flexible, learn to interact differently.

- Find a support system. There are many out there who have been on your road, but each journey is different. Learn from others experiences.

- Feelings and memories, good and bad can intensify during caregiving. Seek out objective opinions from counselors or the Alzheimer's Association.

Take turns with family and friends to avoid burnout

No one can do it all, and the family member or friend who thinks they can, usually ends up in the hospital. Asking for help is a sign of strength! Studies say a high percentage of caregivers die first!

Symptoms of caregiver stress

1. Denial about the disease and its effect on the person who is diagnosed.

2. Anger at the person with dementia, and others who don't understand the disease and frustration that no cure exists!

3. Social withdrawal from friends and activities you once enjoyed. You have to "fill" your boat sometimes. Be realistic. Maybe it is time for more care than you can provide.

4. Anxiety about what lies ahead. No one knows what lies ahead everyone only gets one day at a time!

5. Depression that becomes overwhelming, affecting your ability to function. There is no easy way to deal with a fatal illness.

6. Exhaustion that comes from thinking you can do it all. Reach out and get help. Respite help is available from the Alzheimer's Association.

7. Irritability that comes with trying to make everyone "happy" resentment at the lack of help from family, and need for "me" time. Give yourself credit, not guilt.

8. Lack of concentration that makes it difficult to perform daily tasks. Make notes to help you remember, which helps everyone focus.

9. Health problems can take their toll, physically and mentally. Caregivers often neglect their own health to spend time taking care of the person with Dementia.

There are lots of ways to get help:

• Ask friends to take Mom to lunch or shopping.

• Use a Respite program (respite means-time off from caregiving). Resources may be available to cover the expense of Adult Day Care for a person with Alzheimer's, to pay for someone to come to the home and do activities with your relative so you can go to the store by yourself, or in some case, the respite money may be needed for a short stay in a nursing home if the immediate caregiver is in need of surgery or some other reason for needing help. Consider Senior Companion programs that are usually a free type of respite. These are older people who will just come and keep your loved one company. (Many have training working with people with Alzheimer's)

- Make caregiving a choice. Everyone is a caregiver, has been a caregiver or will need a caregiver. If you make it a choice it can help with resentment about what you are doing!

- Join a support group. Learn from others who have had similar experiences.

Learn as much as you can about the disease.

- Be knowledgeable about medications available and side effects of the current ones.

- Be aware of symptoms just mentioned.

- Every day is different.

- Be realistic about what you are able and willing to do.

- What worked to divert behavior this morning, isn't working now.

- Anticipate problems

- Large groups of people talking can be overwhelming.

- Try small intimate restaurants.

- Watch the news and internet for research about drugs and caregiving. (Caregiving.com and Alzheimer's and Dementia Weekly to name a few)

- Your "attitude" affects your day.

- Some days the Dragon wins!

Coping effectively

Caregiving involves skills we may not have. Unlike some jobs or problems, there is more than one solution and the solutions may need to be different every day! People skills you use in a job and at home are still useful. Choose your battles, maybe it doesn't matter what mom wears, but it DOES matter that she takes her medicine. Learn from others who have struggled, the mothers whose child died of cancer, the young widow whose spouse just died in war, the man whose wife died suddenly in car accident. Their journey and battles are different, but they grieve and go on as you must do. Dare to try new methods in an old relationship. Dad may have always been an "angry" old man, but maybe it is worse now because he is in pain. Don't assume it is the disease, or his personality, sometimes it is the "pain" of age that makes us mad at the world! Try a new approach.

Most caregivers are rookies untrained, uneducated and overwhelmed. Few volunteered for the job, and most are too busy to do one more thing. But you know what they say about getting something done, ask a" busy" person. There is nothing like on-the-job training. Know your limitations. Not everyone can be a caregiver due to the emotional, physical, or financial burdens. Sometimes proximity to your loved one, determines what you can do. Offer to help with finances, phone calls, doctor visits, research into facilities, or home care. If you must find alternative living for the person with dementia, make sure it is a choice you and your family can live with and serve the best interest of your loved one.

Caregiving can be a rewarding, scary, exhausting, sad, frustrating, and funny, all in one day! "Showing up" each day; the happy days and angry days is part of caregiving.

Sibling battles

Sometimes it is easiest to be an only child, where all the decisions are yours. But it is lonely and often you may second-guess your decisions. For the rest of us who have siblings it can also be fraught with problems. Usually siblings have spent a fair amount of their childhood or adulthood bickering about something. Misunderstandings often come between the main caregiver and the brothers or sisters who only come for visits. Sometimes these visits are helpful and may even involve respite for the "hands-on" child or they can be full of judgment, denial about the condition of the parent, excuses why they can't help, and lots of ideas about how to do it better!

Long distance siblings may offer to help, but never be available; want to be praised for the 10 minute phone call to mom; not help with financial expenses; always brag about their vacation when the caregiver hasn't had a whole day off in years; drop in to visit and expect to be entertained; ignore the exhaustion of the "hands-on" sibling; criticize without offering a constructive alternative and may use "Mom liked you best" card to excuse their involvement in the caregiving!

Encourage siblings to be part of the solution, not part of the problem!

My thoughts:

The buck often stops with the caregiver, financially they are in charge, physically they must put their life on hold to help, and emotionally they have the most invested. May it be of comfort to caregivers, that someday hopefully someone will do the same for them.

CHAPTER 10

Children understanding dementia

Children can be people whose parents have a form or dementia, they can be teenagers whose parent has "young onset" dementia, or they can be grandchildren.

Children are greatly affected if you bring home the person who is confused to live with you. Always remember that all this time you are spending taking care of someone with a disease, is time away from them! Time you used spend at their ballgames, listening to stories about school, or just a bedtime story. They may begin to have stomachaches, headaches, or fatigue just to get your attention. Start with information:

- No Grandma is not "crazy", she has a disease. Just like any other disease, but with different symptoms that affect her mind.

- It is not your fault, we aren't sure what causes it, but she isn't contagious.

- We don't know what will happen next, but each day with them is precious! If we can make them laugh, we all will have great memories!

- Are they going to die? Unfortunately, we all die. We don't know when for any of us. But I hope you will enjoy some good days with Grandma, and know that some days she may be more confused and upset. You have good and bad days with friends and at school too.

- Sometimes when it is too hard, sad, or depressing to see the Grandparent they love in this condition. Give them a break.

My thoughts:

As we begin caregiving, we lose sight of our physical and emotional turmoil and its effect on our children. When I was grieving for my Father and caring for my Mother, I didn't realize how hard it was on my children to see me so upset. They can't imagine walking in my shoes, and needed confirmation that their world will still be okay.

CHAPTER 11

Is it time to place them in a facility?

This is truly the million dollar question! We all want people we love as well as ourselves, to live or die at home. But sometimes it is not appropriate for their health, safety, socialization or the disease. Sometimes it isn't about the person with dementia, but the spouse who now has become the 24/7 caregiver. Usually there is a short time when the person with dementia have many physical skills like cooking, laundry or cleaning, but need someone to cognitively keep them on track to do these things. Maybe a woman with dementia can remember what ingredients are for a casserole, but doesn't know whether to cook it on the stove, microwave or oven.

The spouse or caregiver may have some physical problems, such as heart disease, lung disease, or a bad knee, but his mind is very clear. He can pay bills and knows how to run the washing machine. Because of his physical health, the stress and physical responsibility of caregiving can make his health deteriorate quickly. Home health agencies can provide cleaning, cooking, and respite services to let the caregiver have some time and family helping out can buy them some time. Few children or spouses are prepared to be 24/7 caregivers. Most have no knowledge of medication, the course of the disease, nurse training about lifting from falls, or behaviors of the disease.

One recent study said today people over the age of 65 have a 1 in 4 chance of spending time in a nursing home.

Sometimes we make promises to never put them in a nursing home. Our promises should include what will give them the best quality of life and to be sure they are safe.

From my experience, many people with Alzheimer's did better in some sort of facility because the socialization helped with the depression of dementia; the three balanced meals a day (that the spouse didn't have to cook) helped with weight loss; having their medication on a regular basis gave it the best chance to work;, and the activities were good for companionship. If they are living alone, there are more reasons to consider moving. I knew a person with dementia who fell and broke her hip and laid there for 3 hours waiting for someone! Can you imagine the pain? Do you think she ever recovered to her former state of health?

Home versus Facility

Consider these issues as you decide about placement:

- Try to convince them to try it for a week. (If they can still cognitively understand) Then stretch it to two or three. Eventually they will adjust to a new environment. You could even try taking them for a meal, and then tell them it is too late to go home and they will need to spend the night. Will they be upset and angry? Maybe. Are they upset and angry at home some days? Probably. People with Alzheimer's usually adjust to moves better earlier in the disease because they can still make friends and adjust to the new environment.

- Is choosing and placing your loved one in a Facility the answer to all the problems? No, because no one takes care of family like family. But most of us by ourselves can't stay awake and alert 24/7 to make sure they haven't wandered out the door, they can find the bathroom, they are drinking enough water, bathing, eating balanced meals, or going to doctor visits. But together with your loving attention and staff at the facilities, you can cover more of the bases.

- Sometimes the caregiver can become so burnt out physically and emotionally they can't make a decision. Many people wonder what others will think of me if I place my loved one in a facility. How will they treat him when I'm not there? I have no friends, social life, my body hurts everywhere from helping lift and move him but I love him, and how can I be away from him? He will be horribly upset if I move him. He would be at the mercy of people who don't love him. Guilt and resentment can cloud a caregiver's judgment.

- If all else fails, families can use legal papers to place their loved one. Be sure you get advice from an elder attorney, if you are considering this.

- Sometimes behavior like agitation, paranoia or anger can put the caregiver's life in danger! Exhaustion can make the caregiver afraid they won't wake up if the person with dementia is wandering at night.

- See the Alzheimer's Association for a complete checklist for "Making the Decision". Some examples include:

  1. Safety issues-burned pans, cigarette burn, or using walkers

  2. Personal Hygiene-bathing

  3. Behaviors-wandering, agitation

  4. Nutrition- weight loss or gain

  5. Financial concerns-miss work due to caregiving, in home care expensive

  6. Caregiving exhaustion- health of other person helping is at risk

  7. In- home care- not working because of cost, person is not willing, or needing respite and household chores.

Never an easy decision

If the person with dementia is your spouse, it can feel like you have failed! You promised in sickness and in health. Older families worry about taking them away from their friends. (How often are their friends visiting now?) Maybe you have been married a long time and how quiet and lonely it would be without them. (I knew a man who was vacuuming EVERY day because it was so quiet without his spouse.) Sometimes the doctor can help make the decision for you. The person with Alzheimer's may fall, lose mobility or have a stroke and go straight from the hospital to a facility. Those are the easy moves, because there is no guilt about "making the decision", because hospital made the decision.

If it is a parent, think of it as a challenge and remember all the challenges they faced when you were a child. Forgive your parent for getting older, sick and putting you in this position. When you place them in a facility, you will have more time and energy to reminisce about all the good times you have shared. When they are in their own home, you may be cleaning for them, cooking, paying bills, and they get very little of your undivided attention! When you go to visit in a facility, you don't have all those other things to do on your mind.

As you are trying to decide what to do, let me paint another picture of life with an Alzheimer's person. The same mom who could juggle laundry, lunches, 5 course meals, pay the bills and be there for hugs now puts clean clothes in the laundry, overfeeds the fish and last week hid a gallon of ice cream in the linens drawer! Sometimes older spouses have trouble, so instead of helping her bathe, he gave her pills!

Let me tell you the story of a 92 years old blind lady about to enter a facility. Every morning she is well dressed and hair fixed. After stopping at the entrance to her new room, she is given a visual description of all the details, she says I Love It!

But you haven't seen it they said. She replied happiness is something you decide on ahead of time. It is not how you arrange the room but how I arrange my mind. I can spend the day recounting the difficulties with my life and body or be thankful for the parts that still work. Each day is a gift and each day I can review the happy memories I have stored away for this time in my life!

Some spouses or parents go willingly to a facility and maybe are too confused to understand. I had a relative who thought everyone there was her cousin, and made friends. Others think they have been locked in prison and become angry and resentful. Make the decision based on the best information you have with input from family that cares and considering the quality of life they will have physically and emotionally. Remember you have made this choice to the best of your ability, just as your parents made choices for you when you were young. Parenting and caregiving is not a perfect science and they is no one right answer.

Choosing types of dementia care

Families choose dementia facilities based on many things: location to spouse and family, word of mouth for a good reputation, costs, past experiences with other family members or because it is new.

Here is a brief general description of common levels of care: Independent Living, Assisted Living, Dementia Care, Residential placement or a facility.

Independent means your loved one can live by themselves with little or no help from others, but may benefit from a close community of others, smaller housing, handicapped accessible, and options for eating or activities in a central nearby location.

Assisted Living usually means they need some help taking pills, bathing, mobility, or finding their way. This facility provides 3 meals a day and may even bring meals to their room if they are sick. Your loved one may benefit from having 3 meals a day, regular medication activities and socialization.

Dementia care is for people who: are having memory issues, often are taking medication for some type of dementia, may have problems related to the symptoms of dementia such as wandering, anger or paranoia, and need activities appropriate for cognitive loss.

Residential Care is professional staff in residential neighborhood. Most homes have 6-8 residents. Staff is there 24/ 7. For some it is a good option because it is a home.

Facility Care is a type of nursing home. It provides more physical care; residents may mostly be in wheel-chairs and cognitively may be very confused. These people need a lot of care.

Some guidelines to consider include:

- **Environment** - should be clean, smells good, lots of light without glare, low noise level, have an activity room, a safe outdoor area and bathrooms easily accessible and identifiable. Floors should be simple to help with depth perception and wallpaper should be used sparingly as it could promote hallu-cinations. My mom thought the paisley border in her room was ghosts coming to get her, and added to her confusion.

- **Staff** - should be trained in understanding and communicating with people with dementia need be to be happy and friendly. The staff ratio should be adequate for dealing with behavior problems and restless residents at night. The same staff should be on the unit as much as possible familiar faces help your loved one feel more at home. Staff should be patient, treat residents with humor, dignity and affection.

- **Programs** - should be geared toward many activities during the day appropriate for people with a type of dementia; they should be for adults with variety for individual interests. Licensed staff should be aware of the side effects of medication for people with dementia. Communication techniques, redirecting and physical needs, should always be considered before more medication! Staff should be skilled using these methods.

- **Security** - make sure the unit is designed to keep residents from leaving unattended; care should be given so that there is not access to hot stoves, chemicals or medications.

- **Important questions** - Can they remain in the facility if they can no longer walk? If death is imminent can they stay until they have passed? Is hospice allowed in their facility? Must they be continent to live there?

Facilities for dementia care usually cost more than a regular facility that mostly provides physical care. Make

sure there is extra staffing, and programs to justify the expense!

If you make the choice to place your loved one in a facility, thoughts to consider; they may not remember you but you remember them, spousal love is often an acceptance of the present, past and future that will be and will not be. Life isn't always about the bad times but making the most of the time you have.

Alzheimer's Request - (author unknown)

Do not ask me to remember

Don't try to make me understand

Let me rest and know you're with me

Kiss my cheek and hold my hand.

I'm confused beyond your concept,

I'm sad and sick and lost.

All I know is that I need you

To be with me at all costs.

Do not scold or curse or cry,

I can't help the way I'm acting,

I can't be different though I try.

Just remember that I need you,

That the best of me is gone

Please don't fail to stand beside me,

Love me 'til my life is done.

My thoughts:

*Most families want their loved want ones to stay in their own home and die there. But not sure that happens for many. As caregivers we need to focus on the **quality of their life**. They may be in their own home but they are losing weight because they can't remember to eat; aren't taking medication properly (that can be expensive) because they can't remember, are walking over piles of papers because they are either beginning to hoard things or can't make a decision of what to do with them, lastly they may become hermits because they can't drive and are angry at others that try to help.*

Even if they don't want to move... maybe there is a better alternative. Often our loved one becomes unable to make a rational choice (one of the symptoms).

There is some research that people who move into some "community" with services sometimes thrive. Someone else is cooking; they get their medication on time and regularly; they have the stimulation and socialization of others (which helps with depression) and caregivers know they are being cared for and safe. How many of us have any medical knowledge to help if they have a stroke, heart attack or fall and can't get up?

As baby boomers we had more than one parent needing help at a time. They lived in different towns. My mom was confused, my mother-in-law needed surgery.

Don't discount one decision to place them over keeping them at home without weighing all the factors.

CHAPTER 12

End of life

When we love or care for someone with a form of dementia we often go through a stage we call "preceptory" grief. That means that we begin to lose the person we knew, even though they are still alive. Maybe it is their sense of humor, or smile or mellow personality that begins to disappear. Later they may not talk and we miss hearing their voice. Unfortunately, Alzheimer's disease takes a person by pieces, usually parts of their mind that doesn't work and eventually makes parts of their body sick, too.

Grief is a universal experience. We usually begin grieving before they actually die. Sometimes my mom was awfully confused and sad. Did I go home and cry for the smart, vivacious, active woman she was? YES.

Feelings of grief are complex because the person is still alive. But we all know that "vacant" stare when no one is home, behind those eyes. We want their suffering to end, but we don't want to live without them. Even when death is imminent, there is no easy way to lose someone we love. There is grief in moving them to a facility because it means they have progressed to another worse stage, never to get better. People with a type of dementia may have good days and bad, may learn to walk better for a time, but they never "get better" to stay. That is why they call it a progressive disease!

No one knows the exact moment they will leave our earth and go to heaven a happy soul. But because of that, we want to make the most of time we have. It has been proven that people in a coma who can't respond, hear us when we talk and read to them. Why wouldn't that apply to people with Alzheimer's? Just because they are in bed and can't talk doesn't mean their subconscious can't hear wonderful memories they made and words of love! Do it now!

Often people who have dementia will have a few hours or days of clarity before they leave this world. My mom began using names of relatives who had been dead for years. Often they will sit up in bed, (and you can't make them lie back down) and talk to "people on the other side". Give them permission "to go" and safe passage. This isn't about your grief now, but letting them die with dignity.

If they are very alert one day and want to talk about dying, let them! There is no sense in ignoring the white elephant in the room. If they ask "Am I dying?" (As my mom did) say: "I don't know, how do you feel?" Many VERY sick people have lasted weeks or months, waiting for the arrival of a child, grandchild or holiday. It is about their time and God's time. Follow their lead.

Family members have to each work out their own relationships with the person who has dementia. There may be old bad memories, but once the person is gone, we all live with what wasn't settled.

As the body begins to slow down to a stop, sometimes they need oxygen or pain killers. My mom wanted to get up every 10 minutes, to go to the bathroom! (I told her the bathrooms in heaven would be pretty and she could go there!) It turns out she had become too weak to empty her bladder. So they put in a catheter and she could relax.

People often want to go home to die. But with people with dementia, they often are not able to voice these needs. The family needs to decide what is best for them.

Music is always a nice touch for someone with dementia. Hearing is the last sense they lose, so play their favorites! Foot rubs, smiles, laughter, kisses, gazing into their eyes, all communicate compassion and love for a life well lived! Hold their hand and "sit a spell" as the story goes.

Many families sit with the person who is sick around the clock, so they don't die alone. But remember there are equally as many stories, of the family that stepped outside the room for coffee for 5minutes, and their loved one died.

After a person with Alzheimer's has died, families often wonder about an autopsy. Recent studies suggest that current methods of diagnosing are 90%-92% accurate. Now if someone needs to know 100% that is what caused death, maybe you should consider an autopsy. But consider, even if you know that, what can you do with that information? Speaking from having a mom, grandmother and aunt who died from this disease, I know I'm at high risk. If any family member died from this you know you are at risk, does the other 8% confirmation change your life? If family still needs to have an autopsy to be "at peace" with the death, do it now. Be sure emotionally and mentally you will all benefit from that knowledge. An Alzheimer's death should teach us to enjoy each day, because we don't know what our future holds.

Encourage caregivers to take time to recover. Studies suggest it takes 3 years for their bodies to heal after the intense physical and emotional caregiving.

My thoughts:

Remember live every day to the fullest. Every minute is a blessing from God. And never forget... The people who make a difference in our lives are not the ones with the most credentials, the most money, or the awards. They are the ones who care for us. Live simply, love seriously, care deeply and speak kindly! Leave the rest to GOD!

CHAPTER 13

Prevention: The next generation

Clients would call me as soon as they had some family member diagnosed with Alzheimer's. Will I get it? Can I prevent it? How soon will I get it? Unfortunately, science has no sure fire way to prevent this disease. There are some ideas that won't hurt us and can make our whole body healthier, but it doesn't mean for sure we won't get it, any more than getting a flu shot guarantees you won't get the flu!

Here are some ideas:

1. **Exercise** - it is good for your body and the brain. It helps maintain good blood flow to the brain as well as encouraging new cell growth.

2. **Eat Healthy** - We often say if it is good for the heart it is good for the brain. High cholesterol may contribute to stroke and brain damage. Low fat, dark vegetables, fruits and food high in antioxidants may help protect brain cells.

3. **Remain Socially Active** - it makes exercise more fun, reduces stress level, and also helps maintain good brain connections.

4. **Mental Activities** - if you like crossword puzzles, Sudoku, Scrabble, word searches or specific computer games for "mental" exercise, make sure you

exercise your brain too. Sometimes when we are physically tired, we forget to stretch our minds too.

5. **Be Aware of Drugs That Can Affect Brain Function** - some medications such as painkillers, antihistamines, antidepressants, or sleeping pills can affect memory function. Diabetes can effect memory so be aware of blood sugar numbers.

6. **Weight Gain/Loss** - can be a symptom of other health concerns, such as thyroid disease or high cholesterol. Both can cause memory loss. Be sure to check physical causes of confusion first.

7. **Alcohol** - can mix with medication to result in memory loss. Know what is OK to mix. Some studies even suggest that red wine is beneficial.

8. **Vitamins- Omega 3** - can help improve mood, depression, prevent heart attacks, certain cancers and relieve symptoms of inflammation from arthritis. Foods containing omega 3 includes walnuts, canola oil, coconut oil, tuna or salmon. Some research thinks this might be helpful.

    Supplements with B Vitamins - Many people suffer from a deficiency of this vitamin. Vitamin B helps the body keep and make the nerves healthy. (A person with low levels of this vitamin may become anemic, which can cause lots of health problems.) Ask your doctor to test your blood for this vitamin, otherwise you may not know. (My mom had "pernicious anemia" due to low Vitamin B; her body could not absorb it normally. She needed shots, but the anemia gave her Peripheral Neuropathy.) Absorption of Vitamin B-12 deceases with age! There are some studies that suggest this vitamin helps control Homocysteine levels, (an amino acid) which may help prevent heart disease, blood clots and Alzheimer's disease. (This vitamin is in meat, eggs and dairy products).

9. **Drink Plenty Of Fluids** - 25% of water consumed goes to help brain function. Stress can cause the brain to dehydrate, making us more irritable and anxious. Dehydration can also cause medications to be more concentrated, or not work properly, altering the way the body metabolizes. Eat fruit or veggies with high water content. There is even some research that coffee can help be a preventive for dementia!

10. **Let Light Shine In-Winter** -, rain, fog, and clouds interfere with our body's ability to absorb sunshine- Vitamin D. There are many articles about how important Vitamin D is to our body health! It makes it work better. Have your blood tested to discover your level. You might be surprised the energy you have if you take a Vitamin D supplement. There are a few places that have enough sunshine every day for our body.

Older people sometimes have Cataracts or Macular Degeneration which may make them uncomfortable in sunshine. Many of us suffer from Seasonal Affective Disorder (SAD), which can contribute to depression, fatigue and lethargy.

There are full spectrum light bulbs which can help the brain. Vitamin D supplements can help, and of course 15 minutes in the sun! Have your doctor check Vitamin D levels to make sure they are normal.

11. **Control Pain** - Pain can interfere with our ability to heal, to function properly, to rest, to think. When we are in pain our blood flows to the place that hurts. It is a vital sign of health, with blood pressure, temperature, heart rate, and respiration. We all know pain can make it hard to think!

    Consider other alternatives to help with pain beside more medication: physical therapy, exercise, weight loss, stretching, meditation, avoiding food that can cause triggers, treating infections like sinus, or sometimes some "me" time can help relax your body and relieve the pain.

12. **Maintain a Positive Attitude** - Life is a lot of what we expect. Happiness enhances our alertness; ability to receive new information; improves our social connections and even expands to those around us. My rule of life is everyone has something! Do you know anyone who doesn't have some health issues, especially as we age? Appreciate the things you have, that each day we get to try again. An attitude of gratitude can help you live longer and better.

13. **Laugh!** - It feels good, it boosts immunity, it makes others feel good and it produces endorphins which

are natural pain killers! It even gets more oxygen to the brain.

14. **Brain Stimulating Exercises** - Keep learning and trying new things. Try a musical instrument, start a new hobby, join a discussion group, cherish time with family and friends, take a class, go dancing, write a story about things important to you, memorize phone numbers and addresses, try something new and different, shop the opposite way in the grocery store. Breathe deeply. Doing familiar things in a new way uses a different part of the brain.

We all worry when we begin to forget appointments or passwords. Our world has become so full of technical phones, I pads, computers, Kindles and emails, that our brains are challenged almost every moment of every day. Everything has a number! (For those of us who are mathematically challenged, it is a real mind problem). Try "memory" tricks to help remember. Use word association to help remember names, be more observational about what people are wearing, say to yourself "I locked the door." All these tricks may help sharpen your memory. Sleep can help make the memories stick in the brain. You know it is harder to remember when you are stressed. Accept that and know you probably aren't getting any form of dementia, but your brain and body are on overload for now.

My thoughts:

No one knows what tomorrow may bring! Make good choices. Exercise your body and brain. Evaluate your priorities.

Put some humor and a smile in each and every day. Mentally ask yourself if this item, experience, or problem will make a difference to your life 5years from now? Concentrate on things that improve the "quality" of your life! We can't control the quantity.

Each day is special

Someone one once told me:

Old age is like a bank account, you withdraw from what you put in!

So, deposit a LOT of happiness and memories.

Deposit good health and experiences.

Make friends and family an important part of your life.

Enjoy the beautiful days of our lives, look around!

Free your heart from hatred, we can't change the past.

Live simply, we come into the world with nothing and we leave that way.

Give more of your time to help others, money if you can, and love to those you care about.

Expect life to go well. No one's life is perfect.

Celebrate your blessings.

CHAPTER 14

Summary

If this book can make just one family's life easier down this journey of Alzheimer's, I have made a difference. I, too, may lose the stories, experiences, ideas, helpful thoughts and guidance I have learned from the Alzheimer's association and my life experiences. So I needed to write this now. I'm pretty sure there may be no cure in my lifetime, but here are some thoughts in writing that hopefully will help each of you on your journey. It was kept short because none of you have time to read long stories; you need ideas to use today!

My Favorite Alzheimer's Books

<u>Coach Broyles' Playbook for Alzheimer's Caregivers: A Practical Tips Guide</u>, by Frank Broyles

<u>Wilfrid Gordon McDonald Partridge</u>, by Mem Fox

<u>Learning to Speak Alzheimer's: A Groundbreaking Approach for Everyone Dealing with the Disease</u> by Joanne Koenig Coste

<u>The Validation Breakthrough</u>, by Naomi Feil

<u>The 36 Hour Day</u>, by Nancy L Mace and Peter V. Rabins

<u>FAQ Alzheimer's Disease Frequently Asked Questions</u>, by Frena Gray-Davidson

The Forgetting. Alzheimer's: Portrait of an Epidemic. by David Shenk

Elder Rage by Jacqueline Marcell

Still Alice, by Dr. Lisa Genova

Alzheimer's Sourcebook for Caregivers by Frena-Gray Davidson

Moving a Relative with Memory Loss: A Family Caregiver's Guide by Laurie White and Beth Spencer

Handbook for Long Distance Caregivers (available at the Alzheimer's Association)

IPhone App: ALZ & DEMENTIA

Websites and other sources:

www.alz.org – Alzheimer's Association. Has a wealth of information where ever you live, with local resources for support groups, informational meetings, and events. It has 24/7 number (1-800-272-3900) for questions about caregiving on weekends and the middle of the night! Website gives information about the disease, research, caregiving, progression of the disease, helpline to answer questions and referral information for doctors, lawyers, and local aging resources.

www.caregiver.com - Good website for tips, online newsletter, book ideas, and nice editorial

www.alzstore.com - this catalog has good products for Alzheimer's people. Respite videos, phone without buttons, manipulative items, fake check books, and activity books.

www.nia.nih.gov/alzheimers - *National Institute of Health has some good information, free booklet and can have research information.*

www.Reminisce.com - *a magazine that comes every other month with articles and pictures of the past*

www.medicare.gov - *a website with ratings for facilities*

www.bathingwithoutabattle.unc.edu/bathing-techniques *ideas for bathing*

Facebook Pages:

Alzheimers Weekly

Alzheimer's Awareness

CPSIA information can be obtained
at www.ICGtesting.com
Printed in the USA
FSOW02n2158030815
9475FS